# DMSO
## HEALING GUIDE

A Practical Handbook for Safe and
Effective Use of Dimethyl Sulfoxide

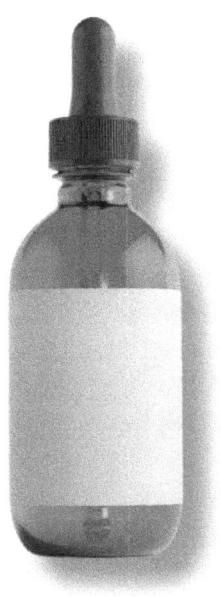

**NICHOLAS GIORDANO**

## Copyright © 2024 Nicholas Giordano

Unauthorized reproduction, distribution, or transmission of any part of this publication in any form or by any means, including photocopying, recording, or other electronic or mechanical methods, without the prior written permission of the publisher, is prohibited. Brief quotations may be used in critical reviews and other non-commercial uses permitted by copyright law, provided proper attribution is given.

# TABLE OF CONTENTS

Part 1: Understanding DMSO ............................................................. 4
CHAPTER ONE ................................................................................ 6
   Introduction to DMSO ................................................................. 6
   How is DMSO used for IC? .......................................................... 8
CHAPTER TWO ............................................................................... 14
   Safety and Usage Guidelines ...................................................... 14
   Grades of DMSO ........................................................................ 14
   Storing and Handling DMSO ...................................................... 16
   Common Side Effects ................................................................. 22
   DMSO Interactions with Medications and Health Conditions . 24
   Why is it essential to talk to your doctor before using DMSO . 25
CHAPTER THREE ............................................................................ 30
   The Science Behind DMSO ........................................................ 30
   DMSO's Ability to Penetrate the Skin affect its Potential Uses 31
   Scientific Research about DMSO's Effectiveness for Various Conditions ................................................................................... 33
Part 2: DMSO and Specific Conditions ............................................. 36
CHAPTER FOUR ............................................................................... 38
   DMSO for Pain and Inflammation .............................................. 38
   Application of DMSO for Pain Relief ........................................ 40
CHAPTER FIVE ................................................................................ 44
   DMSO and Skin Conditions ....................................................... 44
   Instructions and Precautions for using DMSO on Skin ............ 47

Can DMSO be Used with Other Skin Treatments or Medications ............................................................................................. 51
CHAPTER SIX ................................................................................ 56
DMSO and Other Ailments ...................................................... 56
DMSO's Mechanisms of Action ............................................... 59
CHAPTER SEVEN .......................................................................... 68
DMSO and Animals ................................................................. 68
Safety Considerations in Using DMSO to Treat Animals ........ 71
Part 3: Maximizing DMSO's Potential ......................................... 76
CHAPTER EIGHT ........................................................................... 78
Combining DMSO with Other Therapies ................................. 78
Specific Combined Therapies ................................................... 80
Complementary Therapies that Might Work Well with DMSO 91
CHAPTER NINE .............................................................................. 98
DMSO and Lifestyle ................................................................. 98
CHAPTER TEN ............................................................................. 102
Conclusion .............................................................................. 102

# Part 1: Understanding DMSO

$$\text{H}_3\text{C}-\underset{\|}{\overset{\overset{\displaystyle O}{\|}}{S}}-\text{CH}_3$$

# CHAPTER ONE
## Introduction to DMSO

DMSO, short for dimethyl sulfoxide, is an organic sulfur compound with the formula $(CH_3)_2SO$. It appears as a colorless liquid at room temperature and is known for its unique properties, particularly its ability to readily penetrate the skin and other biological membranes. This characteristic has made it a subject of interest in various fields, from medicine to industrial applications.

DMSO is a byproduct of the paper-making process. To understand its origin, we need to talk briefly into how paper is produced. Paper is made from wood pulp, which contains cellulose fibers. These fibers are bound together by a substance called lignin. During the paper-making process, lignin is removed from the wood pulp to produce the desired quality of paper. This extracted lignin undergoes a series of chemical reactions, one of which results in the production of DMSO.

In its pure form, DMSO is odorless. However, it's often associated with a distinctive garlicky odor. This odor is actually attributed to a breakdown product of DMSO, dimethyl sulfide (DMS), which is produced when DMSO comes into contact with certain enzymes in the body.

The discovery of DMSO dates back to the mid-19th century. In 1866, a Russian scientist named Alexander Saytzeff first synthesized this intriguing compound. However, it remained largely a laboratory curiosity for nearly a century.

In the 1960s, DMSO's potential medical applications began to garner attention. Dr. Stanley Jacob, a physician at the Oregon Health Sciences University, stumbled upon its remarkable ability to penetrate tissues and carry other substances along with it.

He observed that applying DMSO to his skin resulted in a rapid and peculiar taste sensation in his mouth—a garlicky flavor. This observation led him to investigate DMSO's properties further.

Dr. Jacob's research sparked a flurry of interest in DMSO's potential therapeutic uses. Early studies suggested that DMSO might have anti-inflammatory properties and could be useful in treating a variety of conditions, from arthritis to skin disorders. Its ability to penetrate the blood-brain barrier also raised hopes for its potential in treating neurological conditions.

However, the initial enthusiasm surrounding DMSO was met with setbacks. Some early clinical trials reported side effects, including skin irritation and eye problems. Concerns were also raised about the purity of DMSO used in some studies, as industrial-grade DMSO could contain impurities that might contribute to adverse effects.

In response to these concerns, the Food and Drug Administration (FDA) in the United States imposed strict regulations on DMSO research and clinical trials. This led to a decline in DMSO's popularity and a period of skepticism surrounding its use.

Despite the regulatory hurdles, research on DMSO continued, albeit at a slower pace. In 1978, the FDA approved DMSO for a specific medical use: the treatment of interstitial cystitis, a painful bladder condition. This approval was based on clinical trials demonstrating its effectiveness in reducing inflammation and pain in the bladder.

In recent years, there has been a renewed interest in DMSO, particularly for its potential in managing pain and inflammation associated with various conditions, such as arthritis and musculoskeletal injuries. However, it's crucial to note that these uses are considered "off-label," meaning they are not officially approved by the FDA.

DMSO's reputation has thus evolved from a laboratory curiosity to a potential wonder drug, then to a subject of controversy, and now to a cautiously explored therapeutic option. While its FDA-approved use remains limited to interstitial cystitis, its unique properties continue to intrigue researchers and clinicians, prompting further investigation into its potential benefits and risks.

While DMSO has garnered a reputation for its potential use in a wide array of health conditions, it's crucial to emphasize that in the United States, the Food and Drug Administration (FDA) has officially approved DMSO for the treatment of only **one** medical condition: **interstitial cystitis**.

Interstitial cystitis (IC), also known as painful bladder syndrome, is a chronic condition that causes bladder pressure, bladder pain, and sometimes pelvic pain. The pain ranges from mild discomfort to severe. The condition can affect both men and women, but it's more common in women.

## How is DMSO used for IC?

DMSO is used in a procedure called **intravesical instillation**, often referred to as a **bladder wash**. This involves a healthcare professional inserting a catheter through the urethra and into the bladder. A DMSO solution is then instilled into the bladder, held for a period of time (usually around 15 minutes), and then drained out.

The exact mechanisms by which DMSO helps with IC are not fully understood, but it is thought to:

- **Reduce inflammation:** DMSO has anti-inflammatory properties, which may help to soothe the irritated bladder lining.

- **Relax the bladder muscles:** This can help to reduce bladder pressure and pain.

- **Increase bladder capacity:** By reducing inflammation and relaxing the muscles, DMSO may allow the bladder to hold more urine.

**Important points to note:**

- **Prescription only:** DMSO for IC is available only by prescription under the brand name Rimso-50.

- **Procedure done by a doctor:** The intravesical instillation procedure must be performed by a qualified healthcare professional.

- **Not a cure:** DMSO is not a cure for IC, but it can help to manage the symptoms.

- **Side effects:** The most common side effect is a garlic-like taste in the mouth and body odor. Other potential side effects include bladder irritation, burning sensation, and mild skin irritation.

DMSO has a curious place in the world of health. While it's only officially approved for one specific condition (interstitial cystitis), there's a buzz around it, with many people intrigued by its potential for a wide range of other ailments. This persistent interest, despite limited official recognition, stems from a fascinating confluence of factors:

**1. DMSO's Unique Properties and Mechanisms:**

- **Unparalleled Penetration:** DMSO has this remarkable ability to cross cell membranes like a ghost, slipping through the skin and into tissues with exceptional ease. This makes it a powerful carrier, potentially enhancing the absorption of other substances.

- Imagine it as a key that unlocks the door for other therapeutic agents to enter the body more effectively. This feature alone fuels speculation about its potential to enhance drug delivery and treat various conditions.

- **Anti-inflammatory Action:** DMSO appears to interfere with the inflammatory process, potentially reducing pain and swelling. Inflammation is a common thread in many health problems, from arthritis to skin injuries, so the idea of a substance that can dampen this fire naturally draws attention.

- **Antioxidant Effects:** Some studies suggest DMSO can scavenge free radicals, those unstable molecules that can damage cells and contribute to various diseases. This antioxidant property adds another layer to its potential therapeutic applications.

- **Analgesic Properties:** DMSO seems to have some pain-relieving effects, possibly by interfering with pain signals or reducing inflammation. For people struggling with chronic pain, the prospect of a different kind of relief is naturally appealing.

## 2. The Power of Anecdotal Evidence:

- **Word-of-Mouth Testimonials:** Many people who have used DMSO for various conditions, even without official approval, report positive experiences. These personal stories, shared through word-of-mouth or online platforms, create a ripple effect of interest. While anecdotal evidence is not a substitute for scientific proof, it can be compelling, especially when traditional treatments have failed.

- **The "Underground" Appeal:** DMSO's somewhat controversial history and its limited official approval, ironically, might contribute to its allure. It can be seen as an "outsider" remedy, a substance that hasn't been fully embraced by the mainstream medical establishment. This can appeal to people who are seeking alternative solutions or who feel disillusioned with conventional treatments.

**3. The Need for More Research:**

- **Gaps in Knowledge:** While some studies have explored DMSO's potential for various conditions, there's still a significant lack of large-scale, rigorous clinical trials to definitively prove its safety and effectiveness beyond interstitial cystitis. This knowledge gap, rather than discouraging interest, fuels curiosity and a desire for further exploration.

- **The Promise of Untapped Potential:** The very fact that DMSO's mechanisms of action are not fully understood leaves room for hope and speculation. It's like a puzzle with missing pieces, and the possibility of unlocking its full therapeutic potential is a tantalizing prospect.

**4. Accessibility and Affordability:**

- **Over-the-Counter Availability:** In some countries, DMSO is readily available without a prescription, making it accessible to people who might be looking for alternative options.

- **Relatively Low Cost:** Compared to many prescription medications, DMSO can be relatively inexpensive, further increasing its appeal, especially for those who are struggling with healthcare costs.

While the interest in DMSO for various health issues is understandable, it's essential to approach its use with caution and a healthy dose of skepticism. The lack of FDA approval for these other uses means that its safety and effectiveness have not been rigorously established. Relying solely on anecdotal evidence can be risky.

# CHAPTER TWO
## Safety and Usage Guidelines
### Grades of DMSO
DMSO is typically categorized into three main grades:

1. **Industrial Grade:** This is the most common and least pure form of DMSO. It's primarily used as a solvent in various industrial processes, such as paint stripping, cleaning, and chemical manufacturing. Industrial-grade DMSO may contain impurities like bacteria, heavy metals, and other chemicals, making it unsuitable and potentially dangerous for human use.

2. **Reagent Grade:** This grade of DMSO is purer than industrial grade and is often used in laboratory settings for research and chemical reactions. While it has fewer impurities, it may still contain trace amounts of contaminants that could be harmful if ingested or applied to the skin.

3. **Pharmaceutical Grade:** This is the purest form of DMSO and the only grade recommended for human use. It meets stringent quality standards set by regulatory bodies like the United States Pharmacopeia (USP) and the European Pharmacopoeia (Ph. Eur.). Pharmaceutical-grade DMSO undergoes rigorous purification processes to remove impurities and ensure safety for medical applications.

### Why Purity Matters
The purity of DMSO is critical for several reasons:

- **Safety:** Impurities in lower-grade DMSO can cause a range of adverse reactions, including skin irritation, allergic reactions, and even more serious health problems if ingested.

Pharmaceutical-grade DMSO is rigorously purified to minimize the risk of such reactions.

- **Effectiveness:** Impurities can interfere with DMSO's therapeutic properties, reducing its effectiveness in treating various conditions. Using the purest form ensures that DMSO can function optimally.

- **Absorption:** DMSO is a highly effective carrier, meaning it can easily penetrate the skin and carry other substances along with it. This property is beneficial for topical applications, but it also means that any impurities present in the DMSO will be absorbed into the body as well. Using pure DMSO minimizes the risk of introducing harmful substances into the bloodstream.

## How to Ensure Purity

- **Look for the USP or Ph. Eur. designation:** When purchasing DMSO, always check the label for the USP or Ph. Eur. designation, which indicates that the product meets pharmaceutical-grade standards.

- **Purchase from reputable sources:** Buy DMSO from reputable suppliers, such as pharmacies or online retailers specializing in health and wellness products. Avoid purchasing from industrial suppliers or unknown sources, as the purity may be questionable.

- **Check the packaging:** Ensure the DMSO is packaged in a sealed, tamper-proof container to prevent contamination.

- **Storage:** Store DMSO in a cool, dark place away from direct sunlight and heat, as these can degrade its quality over time.

By understanding the different grades of DMSO and prioritizing purity, you can ensure safe and effective use for its various potential applications.

Remember, using pharmaceutical-grade DMSO is essential for minimizing risks and maximizing the potential benefits of this versatile compound.

## Storing and Handling DMSO

Storing and handling DMSO properly is crucial not only for preserving its effectiveness but also for ensuring your safety. DMSO is a powerful solvent with unique properties, and a little carelessness can lead to unwanted consequences. Here's a detailed guide to help you store and handle DMSO responsibly:

### Choosing the Right Container

- **Pharmaceutical Grade:** First and foremost, always make sure you're using pharmaceutical-grade DMSO. This grade is specifically purified for medical use and minimizes the risk of contaminants.

- **Glass or HDPE:** DMSO can react with some plastics, so it's best to store it in glass containers or high-density polyethylene (HDPE) plastic containers. These materials are less likely to leach chemicals into the DMSO or be degraded by it.

- **Amber or Dark Glass:** Light can degrade DMSO over time, so amber or dark-colored glass bottles are ideal for storage. If you're using a clear glass container, be sure to store it in a dark place.

- **Airtight Seal:** DMSO readily absorbs moisture from the air, which can dilute it and reduce its effectiveness. Always ensure the container is tightly sealed to prevent this.

### Storage Best Practices

- **Cool, Dark Place:** Store DMSO in a cool, dark place away from direct sunlight and heat sources. A cupboard or cabinet away from appliances that generate heat is a good option.

- **Temperature Considerations:** Ideally, store DMSO at room temperature (around 20-25°C or 68-77°F). Avoid storing it in the refrigerator, as it can solidify at lower temperatures (around 18.5°C or 65.3°F). If it does solidify, you can gently warm it to room temperature to return it to its liquid state. Never use a microwave or direct heat to thaw DMSO.

- **Keep Away from Children and Pets:** Like any chemical substance, store DMSO out of reach of children and pets to prevent accidental ingestion or contact.

- **Label Clearly:** Always label the container clearly with "DMSO" and the date of purchase. This helps prevent confusion and ensures you know how long you've had it.

### Handling Precautions

- **Gloves:** When handling DMSO, especially for topical applications, wear gloves to prevent skin irritation or absorption of other substances through the DMSO. Nitrile gloves are a good choice.

- **Avoid Spills:** DMSO can easily penetrate clothing and skin. Be careful not to spill it. If you do, clean it up immediately with water.

- **Eye Protection:** If there's a risk of splashing, wear eye protection.

- **Wash Hands:** Always wash your hands thoroughly after handling DMSO, even if you've worn gloves.

- **Don't Mix with Other Chemicals:** Unless specifically instructed by a healthcare professional, avoid mixing DMSO with other chemicals, as this can create unpredictable reactions or byproducts.

- **Application:** When applying DMSO topically, use a clean cotton ball or applicator. Avoid using your bare hands to apply it.

- **Concentration:** For topical use, DMSO is often diluted with water. Always follow the recommended dilution guidelines provided by your healthcare professional or in reputable sources.

## Ways DMSO can be Applied or Used?

DMSO is a versatile substance with a range of applications, thanks in large part to its unique ability to penetrate the skin and other biological membranes. However, it's crucial to remember that only one application is officially approved by the FDA: the treatment of interstitial cystitis (a painful bladder condition). All other uses are considered "off-label" and haven't undergone the same rigorous testing for safety and effectiveness.

Here's a breakdown of the various ways DMSO can be applied or used, with important caveats:

### 1. Topical Application

This is the most common way people use DMSO. It involves applying it directly to the skin, often in a diluted form (typically with water or a carrier oil).

- **Purposes:**
  - **Pain relief:** People apply it to areas affected by arthritis, muscle strains, sprains, and other types of musculoskeletal pain.
  - **Inflammation reduction:** It may help reduce inflammation in conditions like tendonitis, bursitis, and skin conditions like eczema.
  - **Wound healing:** Some believe it can promote faster healing of cuts, burns, and skin ulcers.
  - **Scar reduction:** There are claims that DMSO can help reduce the appearance of scars.
  - **Skin conditions:** It's sometimes used for conditions like psoriasis, scleroderma, and shingles.
- **Important Considerations:**
  - **Dilution:** Always dilute DMSO before applying it to the skin. Common dilutions range from 50% to 90% DMSO, with the rest being water or a carrier oil.
  - **Skin sensitivity:** DMSO can cause skin irritation or allergic reactions in some people. It's a good idea to do a patch test on a small area of skin before applying it more widely.
  - **Clean skin:** Apply DMSO to clean, dry skin. Avoid applying it to broken or irritated skin.
  - **Absorption:** DMSO can increase the absorption of other substances through the skin. Be cautious about what other products you use on the same area.

## 2. Transdermal Application

This involves using DMSO as a carrier to enhance the absorption of other substances through the skin.

- **Purposes:**
    - **Drug delivery:** DMSO can be mixed with certain medications to help them penetrate the skin more effectively. This is sometimes used for pain relief, anti-inflammatory effects, or delivering medications to deeper tissues.
    - **Nutrient absorption:** Some people use DMSO to enhance the absorption of vitamins, minerals, or other nutrients applied topically.
- **Important Considerations:**
    - **Medical supervision:** Using DMSO for transdermal drug delivery should only be done under the guidance of a healthcare professional.
    - **Drug interactions:** DMSO can interact with certain medications. It's essential to consult a doctor before combining it with any other medications.

## 3. Instillation

This method involves a healthcare professional instilling DMSO directly into the bladder.

- **Purpose:**
    - **Interstitial cystitis:** This is the only FDA-approved use of DMSO. It helps relieve the pain and inflammation associated with this condition.

- **Important Considerations:**
  - **Medical procedure:** This procedure should only be performed by a qualified healthcare professional.

## 4. Intravenous Administration

In some cases, DMSO may be administered intravenously, but this is generally limited to specific medical settings and under strict supervision.

- **Purposes:**
  - **Amyloidosis:** DMSO is sometimes used intravenously to treat amyloidosis, a condition where abnormal proteins build up in organs and tissues.
  - **Brain swelling:** It may be used in emergency situations to reduce swelling in the brain after a head injury.
- **Important Considerations:**
  - **Hospital setting:** Intravenous DMSO administration should only be done in a hospital setting under the care of a medical professional.
  - **Serious risks:** This method carries a higher risk of side effects and complications.

## 5. Other Uses

- **Veterinary medicine:** DMSO is sometimes used in veterinary medicine for similar purposes as in humans, such as pain relief, inflammation reduction, and wound healing.
- **Industrial solvent:** DMSO is a powerful solvent used in various industrial applications, such as paint thinners, cleaning agents, and in the manufacturing of electronics.

However, industrial-grade DMSO should never be used for medicinal purposes.

## **Common Side Effects**

- **Garlic-like Taste and Odor:** This is the most common side effect, occurring due to a metabolite of DMSO called dimethyl sulfide. It can cause a garlic-like taste in the mouth and a distinct body odor that can linger for a few days.
    - **What to do:** While generally harmless, this can be unpleasant. Staying hydrated, practicing good oral hygiene, and showering regularly can help manage the odor.

- **Skin Reactions:** Topical application can cause skin irritation, redness, itching, burning, dryness, or scaling in some people. In rare cases, blistering or allergic reactions can occur.
    - **What to do:** Discontinue use immediately and wash the affected area with mild soap and water. If irritation persists or is severe, consult a doctor. Consider diluting DMSO further for future applications.

- **Gastrointestinal Issues:** If ingested, DMSO can cause nausea, vomiting, diarrhea, or constipation.
    - **What to do:** If you experience these symptoms after ingesting DMSO, discontinue use and consult a

doctor. Stay hydrated to prevent dehydration from vomiting or diarrhea.

- **Headache and Dizziness:** Some people may experience headaches or dizziness, especially with higher concentrations or prolonged use.
    - **What to do:** If you experience these symptoms, stop using DMSO and rest. If they persist or become severe, seek medical advice.

- **Other Potential Side Effects:** Less common side effects include drowsiness, changes in vision, and allergic reactions (such as hives or difficulty breathing).

## What to Do if Side Effects Occur

- **Discontinue Use:** The first step is to stop using DMSO immediately.

- **Wash Affected Area:** If you experience skin irritation, wash the area thoroughly with mild soap and water.

- **Hydrate:** Drink plenty of water, especially if you experience gastrointestinal issues or headache.

- **Seek Medical Advice:** If side effects are severe, persistent, or concerning, consult a doctor or healthcare professional.

- **Document Your Experience:** Keep track of any side effects you experience, including when they occurred, their severity, and how long they lasted. This information can be helpful for your doctor.

# DMSO Interactions with Medications and Health Conditions

DMSO can interact with certain medications and may be contraindicated in some health conditions. It's crucial to be aware of these potential interactions:

## Medications

- **Blood Thinners:** DMSO may increase the effects of blood thinners, such as warfarin (Coumadin), potentially increasing the risk of bleeding.

- **Sedatives:** DMSO may enhance the sedative effects of medications like benzodiazepines or barbiturates.

- **Steroids:** DMSO may increase the absorption and effects of topical steroids.

- **Other Medications:** DMSO can potentially interact with a variety of other medications. It's essential to discuss any medications you're taking with your doctor before using DMSO.

## Health Conditions

- **Liver or Kidney Problems:** DMSO is primarily metabolized by the liver and excreted by the kidneys. People with liver or kidney disease should use DMSO with caution, as it may put extra stress on these organs.

- **Diabetes:** DMSO may affect blood sugar levels, so individuals with diabetes should monitor their blood sugar closely when using DMSO.

- **Pregnancy and Breastfeeding:** The safety of DMSO during pregnancy and breastfeeding has not been well established. It's best to avoid using DMSO during these times.

- **Eye Conditions:** DMSO can penetrate the eyes. People with glaucoma or other eye conditions should use caution when applying DMSO near the eyes.

## Why is it essential to talk to your doctor before using DMSO

Even though DMSO might seem like a simple, natural remedy, it's absolutely crucial to talk to your doctor before using it, even for seemingly minor health issues. Here's why:

### 1. DMSO's Powerful Solvent Properties:

DMSO is a highly effective solvent, meaning it can dissolve many substances. This property, while beneficial for some applications, also means it can easily carry other substances across your skin and into your bloodstream. This can be problematic if:

- **You're using impure DMSO:** If your DMSO contains impurities (which is possible with industrial-grade DMSO), those impurities can be absorbed into your body, potentially causing harm.

- **You're using other topical medications:** DMSO can increase the absorption of other medications applied to your skin, leading to unintended and possibly dangerous increases in their effects.

### 2. Potential Side Effects and Reactions:

While generally considered safe when used correctly, DMSO can cause side effects, including:

- **Skin irritation:** Redness, itching, burning, or dryness at the application site.

- **Allergic reactions:** Some people may experience allergic reactions to DMSO, which can range from mild skin rashes to more serious systemic reactions.
- **Gastrointestinal issues:** Nausea, vomiting, or diarrhea, especially if DMSO is ingested.
- **Strong body odor:** A garlic-like odor on the breath and skin is a common side effect, which can be unpleasant and persistent.

Your doctor can help you assess your risk for these side effects and advise you on how to minimize them.

## 3. Drug Interactions:

DMSO can interact with certain medications, potentially increasing or decreasing their effectiveness or causing other adverse reactions. Some medications that may interact with DMSO include:

- **Blood thinners:** DMSO may increase the risk of bleeding when used with blood thinners like warfarin (Coumadin).
- **Sedatives:** DMSO may enhance the effects of sedatives, leading to excessive drowsiness.
- **Steroids:** DMSO may increase the absorption of steroids, potentially leading to increased side effects.
- **Chemotherapy drugs:** DMSO may interfere with the effectiveness of certain chemotherapy medications.

Your doctor can review your medication list and identify any potential interactions with DMSO.

### 4. Underlying Health Conditions:

Certain health conditions may make using DMSO risky. For example:

- **Liver or kidney problems:** These organs are involved in metabolizing and eliminating DMSO, so existing problems could be exacerbated.
- **Diabetes:** DMSO may affect blood sugar levels.
- **Pregnancy or breastfeeding:** The safety of DMSO during pregnancy or breastfeeding is not well established.

Your doctor can assess your overall health and advise you on whether DMSO is safe for you to use.

### 5. Proper Usage and Dosage:

Your doctor can provide guidance on the appropriate way to use DMSO for your specific situation, including:

- **Concentration:** DMSO is often diluted before topical application. Your doctor can recommend the correct concentration.
- **Application method:** There are different ways to apply DMSO (e.g., directly to the skin, with a compress, etc.). Your doctor can advise on the best method for your needs.
- **Frequency and duration:** Your doctor can tell you how often to use DMSO and for how long.
- 

### 6. Monitoring and Adjustments:

Even if your doctor gives you the green light to use DMSO, it's important to keep them informed about your experience.

Let your doctor know if you experience any side effects or if your condition doesn't improve. They may need to adjust your treatment plan or recommend alternative therapies.

# CHAPTER THREE
## The Science Behind DMSO

DMSO, or dimethyl sulfoxide, is a fascinating molecule with a somewhat enigmatic mechanism of action. While we don't have a complete picture of how it works its magic within the body, we do know enough to understand some of its key effects on a scientific level.

One of the most remarkable characteristics of DMSO is its ability to readily cross cell membranes, including the skin barrier. This unique property is attributed to its amphipathic nature, meaning it has both polar and nonpolar characteristics.

This allows it to interact with both water-loving and water-fearing molecules, making it a versatile solvent and enabling it to penetrate tissues easily. This rapid penetration is why DMSO is often used as a carrier to enhance the absorption of other substances through the skin.

Once inside the body, DMSO exerts a variety of effects. One of its primary mechanisms is believed to be its anti-inflammatory action. It appears to achieve this by several pathways. DMSO can scavenge free radicals, those unstable molecules that can damage cells and contribute to inflammation. It also seems to inhibit the production of inflammatory cytokines, which are signaling molecules that promote inflammation. Furthermore, DMSO may alter the behavior of white blood cells, reducing their migration to sites of inflammation.

DMSO also demonstrates analgesic, or pain-relieving, properties. It's thought to achieve this by blocking nerve conduction fibers that transmit pain signals. In essence, it may be interrupting the communication of pain messages to the brain.

This effect, combined with its anti-inflammatory action, could explain why some people find DMSO helpful for conditions like arthritis and muscle injuries.

Beyond these primary mechanisms, DMSO may also influence the immune system. Some studies suggest it can modulate immune responses, potentially making it useful in managing autoimmune conditions where the body's immune system mistakenly attacks its own tissues. However, more research is needed to fully understand DMSO's role in immune modulation.

Another interesting aspect of DMSO is its potential to affect cellular processes. It appears to influence cell differentiation, which is the process by which cells become specialized. This has led to investigations into its possible use in cancer treatment, although this remains a controversial area with much more research needed.

It's important to note that despite these known mechanisms, DMSO's full range of actions in the body is still being explored. There may be other subtle ways it interacts with cells and tissues that we don't yet fully comprehend. This complexity is partly what makes DMSO such an intriguing molecule and why research into its potential continues.

## **DMSO's Ability to Penetrate the Skin affect its Potential Uses**

DMSO's remarkable ability to penetrate the skin is a key factor driving its diverse range of potential applications. Unlike many other substances that struggle to cross the skin's protective barrier, DMSO readily passes through, carrying other compounds along with it. This unique characteristic opens up exciting possibilities in various fields, from pain management to drug delivery.

One of the most significant implications of DMSO's skin penetration ability is its potential to enhance the delivery of topical medications. Imagine applying a cream or ointment to your skin, only to have most of it sit on the surface, unable to reach the underlying tissues where it's needed.

DMSO can change that. By acting as a carrier, it can help transport these medications through the skin barrier and into the deeper layers, potentially increasing their effectiveness and reducing the need for oral or injected drugs. This is particularly valuable for conditions like arthritis, where localized pain and inflammation can be targeted directly.

DMSO's ability to penetrate the skin allows it to act as more than just a carrier. It can also exert its own effects within the body. Studies suggest that DMSO may have anti-inflammatory and analgesic properties, meaning it can help reduce pain and swelling. When applied topically, it can potentially reach affected tissues directly, offering a localized approach to pain relief. This is why some people use DMSO for conditions like muscle strains, sprains, and even nerve pain.

Beyond pain management, DMSO's skin penetration has implications for treating various skin conditions. Its ability to carry other substances through the skin barrier makes it a valuable tool for delivering medications directly to the site of skin infections, wounds, or burns.

This targeted approach can potentially enhance healing and reduce the risk of complications. Moreover, some researchers believe that DMSO itself may have properties that promote wound healing and tissue regeneration, although more research is needed to confirm these effects.

However, it's important to acknowledge that DMSO's skin penetration ability also comes with potential risks.

Because it can carry other substances along with it, there's a concern that it could inadvertently transport harmful chemicals or toxins into the body. This is why it's crucial to use only pharmaceutical-grade DMSO and to avoid applying it to areas with broken or damaged skin.

Additionally, DMSO can interact with certain medications, so it's essential to consult with a healthcare professional before using it, especially if you're taking any other drugs.

DMSO's ability to penetrate the skin is a double-edged sword. It offers exciting possibilities for enhancing drug delivery, providing localized pain relief, and treating skin conditions.

However, it's essential to use DMSO responsibly and under the guidance of a healthcare professional to minimize any potential risks. As research continues to explore the full extent of DMSO's capabilities, we can expect to see even more innovative applications emerge in the future.

## **Scientific Research about DMSO's Effectiveness for Various Conditions**

While DMSO has garnered significant attention for its potential therapeutic applications across a wide range of conditions, the scientific evidence supporting its effectiveness is somewhat mixed and often inconclusive. This is partly due to the limited number of rigorous, well-controlled studies and the challenges in conducting research on a substance with such diverse purported uses.

*Here's a breakdown of what research does and doesn't tell us about DMSO's effectiveness for various conditions:*

## Conditions with Some Evidence of Effectiveness

- **Interstitial Cystitis:** This is the only condition for which DMSO has received FDA approval in the United States. Studies have shown that DMSO instilled directly into the bladder can help relieve pain, frequency, and urgency associated with interstitial cystitis. The exact mechanisms are not fully understood, but it's thought that DMSO may reduce inflammation, relax the bladder muscles, and act as a scavenger of free radicals.

- **Musculoskeletal Pain:** Some studies suggest that topical DMSO may provide short-term pain relief for conditions like arthritis, sprains, and strains. It's believed that DMSO may work by reducing inflammation, inhibiting pain signals, and increasing blood flow to the affected area. However, the evidence is not robust, and more high-quality studies are needed to confirm these findings.

- **Skin Conditions:** There's some evidence that DMSO may promote wound healing and reduce scar formation. It may also be helpful in treating certain skin conditions like scleroderma and shingles. However, research in this area is limited, and the mechanisms are not fully elucidated.

## Conditions with Limited or Conflicting Evidence

- **Neurological Conditions:** DMSO has been explored as a potential treatment for neurological conditions like stroke, spinal cord injury, and multiple sclerosis. While some animal studies and small clinical trials have shown promising results, larger and more rigorous studies are needed to determine its true effectiveness and safety in humans.

- **Cancer:** The use of DMSO in cancer treatment is highly controversial. While some proponents claim that DMSO can shrink tumors or enhance the effects of chemotherapy, there's no strong scientific evidence to support these claims. The American Cancer Society cautions against using DMSO for cancer treatment, as it may delay or interfere with proven therapies.

- **Mental Health Conditions:** There have been claims that DMSO can help with mental health conditions like depression and anxiety, but there's no reliable scientific evidence to back up these claims.

Despite the limitations of current research, DMSO remains a promising therapeutic agent with the potential to benefit various conditions. Further research, particularly large, well-controlled clinical trials, is needed to clarify its effectiveness and safety.

It's crucial to approach claims about DMSO's benefits with a healthy dose of skepticism and rely on evidence-based information from reputable sources. Consulting with a healthcare professional is always recommended before using DMSO for any health condition.

# Part 2: DMSO and Specific Conditions

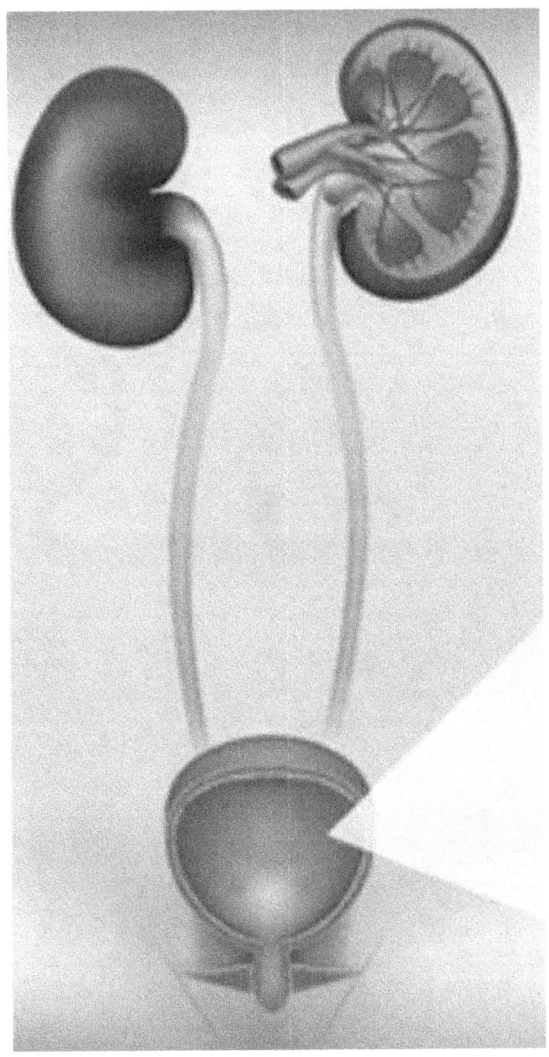

# CHAPTER FOUR
## **DMSO for Pain and Inflammation**

While DMSO is not FDA-approved for a wide range of pain and inflammation conditions, it has garnered significant interest for its potential to alleviate discomfort in various scenarios. It's crucial to remember that evidence for these applications is often anecdotal or based on limited studies, and consulting with a healthcare professional before using DMSO for any health issue is vital.

That being said, let's explore the types of pain and inflammation where DMSO has shown some promise:

### Musculoskeletal Pain

This is a broad category encompassing pain originating from muscles, bones, and joints. Many people turn to DMSO for relief from:

- **Arthritis:** Both osteoarthritis (wear-and-tear arthritis) and rheumatoid arthritis (an autoimmune condition) involve joint inflammation and pain. Some users report that topical DMSO applications can reduce stiffness and discomfort.

- **Muscle strains and sprains:** DMSO may help soothe sore muscles and promote healing after injuries like strains and sprains.

- **Back pain:** Whether it's from muscle tension, a slipped disc, or other spinal issues, DMSO is sometimes used to manage chronic back pain.

- **Tendinitis and bursitis:** These conditions involve inflammation of the tendons and bursae (fluid-filled sacs that cushion joints), respectively. DMSO may help reduce inflammation and pain in these areas.

### Nerve-Related Pain

DMSO has also been explored for its potential to alleviate nerve-related pain, including:

- **Neuropathy:** This refers to nerve damage that can cause numbness, tingling, and pain, often in the hands and feet. Some individuals with diabetic neuropathy or other forms of neuropathy find DMSO helpful in managing their symptoms.

- **Shingles pain:** Shingles is a viral infection that can cause a painful rash and lingering nerve pain (postherpetic neuralgia). DMSO is sometimes used topically to reduce this pain.

- **Complex regional pain syndrome (CRPS):** This is a chronic pain condition that often affects a limb after an injury. Limited evidence suggests that DMSO might be beneficial in managing CRPS symptoms.

DMSO has been used anecdotally for a variety of other painful conditions, such as:

- **Headaches:** Some individuals apply DMSO topically to their temples or forehead to relieve headaches, including migraines.

- **Inflammation from injuries:** DMSO may help reduce swelling and pain associated with various injuries, including bruises, sprains, and fractures.

- **Scar tissue pain:** DMSO is sometimes used to soften scar tissue and reduce associated pain and discomfort.

- **Inflammatory skin conditions:** While DMSO is not a primary treatment for skin conditions, it may help reduce inflammation associated with eczema, psoriasis, and other skin issues.

While DMSO holds promise for managing various types of pain and inflammation, it's essential to approach its use with caution and informed decision-making.

## Application of DMSO for Pain Relief

When it comes to using DMSO for pain relief, proper application and dosage are essential. While DMSO can be a powerful tool, it's important to treat it with respect and follow guidelines to maximize its potential benefits while minimizing any risks. Here's a breakdown of how to apply DMSO for pain, along with dosage considerations:

### Methods of Application

DMSO is most commonly applied topically to the skin. Here are the typical methods:

- **Direct Application:** Apply a small amount of DMSO directly to the affected area using a clean cotton ball, gauze pad, or applicator. Gently rub it into the skin until it's absorbed.

- **Compresses:** Soak a clean cloth in a diluted DMSO solution and apply it as a compress to the painful area. Cover the compress with plastic wrap to prevent evaporation and hold it in place with a bandage or wrap.

- **Gel or Cream:** DMSO is also available in gel or cream formulations, which can be easier to apply and less messy than liquid DMSO. Follow the product instructions for application.

**Dosage Considerations**

There's no one-size-fits-all dosage for DMSO. The amount you use will depend on several factors, including:

- **Concentration:** DMSO is often diluted with water for topical use. Common concentrations range from 50% to 90%. Higher concentrations may be more effective but also increase the risk of skin irritation.

- **Size of the Affected Area:** Larger areas may require more DMSO.

- **Severity of Pain:** More severe pain may warrant a higher concentration or more frequent applications.

- **Individual Sensitivity:** People react differently to DMSO. Start with a lower concentration and gradually increase it as needed, while monitoring for any adverse reactions.

**General Guidelines**

While specific dosage recommendations can vary, here are some general guidelines to get you started:

- **Start Low, Go Slow:** Begin with a lower concentration (e.g., 50%) and apply a small amount to a small area to test your skin's sensitivity.

- **Gradual Increase:** If you tolerate it well, you can gradually increase the concentration or the amount applied, as needed.

- **Frequency:** Apply DMSO 1-3 times per day, or as directed by your healthcare professional.

- **Duration:** The duration of treatment will depend on the condition and your response. For chronic pain, you may need to use DMSO long-term, but always consult your doctor for guidance.

While DMSO is not FDA-approved for pain relief outside of interstitial cystitis, there are numerous anecdotal accounts and some documented cases suggesting its potential in this area. It's important to approach these with a balanced perspective, acknowledging the lack of rigorous scientific backing while recognizing the experiences of those who have used DMSO for pain.

Online forums and communities dedicated to alternative therapies are filled with personal stories from individuals who claim to have found relief from various types of pain using DMSO. These accounts often describe its use for:

- **Arthritis:** Many people report reduced joint pain and stiffness, particularly in conditions like osteoarthritis. They often describe applying DMSO topically to the affected joints, sometimes in combination with other natural remedies.

- **Muscle injuries:** Athletes and those with muscle strains or sprains often share their experiences of using DMSO to reduce pain and inflammation, potentially speeding up recovery time.

- **Neuropathic pain:** Some individuals with nerve-related pain, such as that caused by shingles or diabetic neuropathy, report finding relief with DMSO.

- **Headaches:** Even for conditions like tension headaches or migraines, some people claim that topical DMSO application to the temples or neck can provide relief.

It's crucial to remember that these are personal testimonials, not scientifically controlled studies. The placebo effect, individual variations in pain perception, and other factors can influence these experiences.

While large-scale clinical trials on DMSO for pain are limited, there are some documented cases and smaller studies that provide glimpses into its potential:

- **A 1965 study:** Published in the journal *Annals of the New York Academy of Sciences*, this study explored the use of DMSO in various conditions, including musculoskeletal pain and inflammation. The researchers observed positive results in some patients, with reduced pain and improved mobility.

- **Case reports:** Medical journals occasionally publish case reports where DMSO has been used, sometimes in combination with other treatments, to manage pain in specific situations. These reports often involve complex cases where conventional treatments have failed.

- **Veterinary medicine:** DMSO is more widely used in veterinary medicine for pain management in animals. This provides some indirect evidence for its potential, though human physiology can differ.

While anecdotal accounts and some documented cases suggest DMSO might have pain-relieving properties, it's essential to approach these with cautious optimism.

More research is needed to confirm its efficacy and establish safe and effective protocols for various types of pain. If you're considering using DMSO for pain, it's crucial to consult with your doctor to discuss the potential benefits and risks, and to ensure it won't interact with any existing medications or health conditions.

# CHAPTER FIVE
## DMSO and Skin Conditions

DMSO has garnered significant attention for its potential to aid in wound healing, alleviate burns, reduce the appearance of scars, and even combat skin infections. While it's crucial to remember that DMSO is not FDA-approved for these uses, exploring the mechanisms and anecdotal evidence surrounding its topical application for skin-related issues can offer valuable insights.

**Wound Healing**

DMSO's potential to promote wound healing stems from several key properties:

- **Anti-inflammatory Action:** DMSO is a potent anti-inflammatory agent. It can reduce swelling, pain, and redness associated with wounds, creating a more conducive environment for healing.

- **Enhanced Blood Flow:** DMSO can increase blood flow to the affected area, delivering essential nutrients and oxygen needed for tissue repair.

- **Free Radical Scavenging:** DMSO acts as a free radical scavenger, neutralizing harmful molecules that can impede the healing process.

- **Collagen Synthesis:** Some studies suggest that DMSO may stimulate collagen production, a crucial protein for skin repair and scar formation.

- **Cellular Regeneration:** DMSO might also promote the growth and regeneration of new cells, accelerating the healing process.

Anecdotal reports and some studies suggest that DMSO may be beneficial for various types of wounds, including:

- **Cuts and Abrasions:** DMSO may help reduce pain and inflammation and speed up the healing of minor cuts and scrapes.

- **Surgical Wounds:** Some individuals use DMSO to aid in the healing of surgical incisions, potentially reducing scarring and discomfort.

- **Ulcers:** DMSO has been explored for its potential to promote the healing of chronic ulcers, such as diabetic foot ulcers and pressure sores.

**Burns**

DMSO's anti-inflammatory and analgesic (pain-relieving) properties make it a potential candidate for burn treatment. It may help:

- **Reduce Pain:** DMSO can significantly reduce the pain associated with burns, offering relief during the healing process.

- **Minimize Inflammation:** By reducing inflammation, DMSO may help prevent further tissue damage and promote faster healing.

- **Improve Blood Circulation:** Enhanced blood flow to the burn area can facilitate the delivery of oxygen and nutrients, aiding in tissue regeneration.

It's important to note that DMSO should only be used on minor burns under the guidance of a healthcare professional. Severe burns require immediate medical attention.

**Scars**

DMSO's ability to penetrate the skin and potentially stimulate collagen production has led to its use in scar management. It may help:

- **Reduce Scar Tissue Formation:** By modulating the inflammatory response and promoting healthy collagen synthesis, DMSO might help minimize the formation of excessive scar tissue.
- **Soften and Flatten Scars:** DMSO may help soften and flatten existing scars, making them less noticeable.
- **Improve Scar Appearance:** Some individuals report that DMSO can improve the color and texture of scars, blending them more seamlessly with the surrounding skin.

While anecdotal evidence suggests that DMSO can be helpful for scar reduction, more research is needed to confirm its effectiveness and establish optimal treatment protocols.

**Skin Infections**

DMSO's ability to penetrate the skin and carry other substances with it has led to its exploration as a potential adjunct in treating skin infections. It may:

- **Enhance Antibiotic Penetration:** When used in conjunction with topical antibiotics, DMSO may help the medication penetrate deeper into the skin, reaching the site of infection more effectively.
- **Reduce Inflammation:** DMSO's anti-inflammatory properties can help alleviate the redness, swelling, and discomfort associated with skin infections.

- **Promote Healing:** By reducing inflammation and potentially enhancing the delivery of antibiotics, DMSO may contribute to faster healing of infected skin.

It's crucial to remember that DMSO should not be used as a substitute for prescribed antibiotics. Always consult a healthcare professional for the proper diagnosis and treatment of skin infections.

## **Instructions and Precautions for using DMSO on Skin**

While DMSO can be a helpful tool for certain skin conditions, it's essential to treat it with respect and follow careful guidelines. Here's a comprehensive look at the precautions and best practices for topical DMSO application:

### 1. Purity and Dilution

- **Pharmaceutical Grade Only:** Always begin with pure, pharmaceutical-grade DMSO. This ensures you're working with a substance free of impurities that could irritate your skin or cause other problems. Never use industrial-grade DMSO, as it may contain contaminants.

- **Dilution is Key:** DMSO is rarely applied to the skin at full strength (100%). It's typically diluted with distilled water to reduce the risk of irritation. Common dilutions range from 50% to 70%, but always follow the guidance of your healthcare professional or a reliable source for the specific condition you're addressing.

### 2. Preparing for Application

- **Cleanse the Area:** Before applying DMSO, thoroughly cleanse the affected area with mild, unscented soap and water. This removes any dirt, oils, or lotions that could interfere with DMSO absorption or cause reactions. Pat the skin dry with a clean towel.

- **Sensitivity Test:** Before applying DMSO to a large area or to sensitive skin, perform a patch test. Apply a small amount of the diluted DMSO solution to a small, inconspicuous area of skin (like the inner forearm). Wait 24 hours and observe for any signs of irritation, such as redness, itching, or burning. If you experience a reaction, discontinue use and consult your healthcare provider.

## 3. Application Techniques

- **Gloves:** Always wear gloves when handling and applying DMSO. This protects your hands from irritation and prevents the transfer of any contaminants to the DMSO or your skin. Nitrile gloves are a good option.

- **Applicators:** Use clean cotton balls, gauze pads, or a soft cloth to apply the DMSO solution. Avoid using your bare hands, as DMSO can carry other substances through the skin.

- **Gentle Application:** Apply the DMSO solution gently to the affected area. Don't rub it in vigorously, as this can irritate the skin.

- **Avoid Sensitive Areas:** Avoid applying DMSO to your eyes, mucous membranes (inside the nose, mouth), or broken skin. If accidental contact occurs, flush the area thoroughly with water.

## 4. Frequency and Duration

- **Follow Recommendations:** The frequency and duration of DMSO applications will vary depending on the condition you're treating and the concentration of the solution. Always follow the guidance of your healthcare provider or a reliable source.

- **Start Slowly:** If you're new to using DMSO, start with a lower concentration and fewer applications per day. Gradually increase the frequency or concentration as tolerated.

- **Observe Your Skin:** Pay close attention to how your skin reacts to DMSO. If you experience any irritation, reduce the frequency of application, dilute the solution further, or discontinue use altogether.

## 5. Post-Application Care

- **Allow to Dry:** After applying DMSO, allow the area to air dry completely. Avoid covering the area with tight clothing or bandages immediately after application, as this can trap heat and increase the risk of irritation.

- **Moisturize (If Needed):** If you experience dryness or irritation, you can apply a gentle, unscented moisturizer to the area after the DMSO has dried.

- **Avoid Sun Exposure:** DMSO can increase the skin's sensitivity to sunlight. Avoid exposing the treated area to direct sunlight for several hours after application. If sun exposure is unavoidable, use sunscreen with an SPF of 30 or higher.

## 6. Potential Side Effects and Reactions

- **Skin Irritation:** The most common side effect of topical DMSO use is skin irritation, which may include redness, itching, burning, or dryness. If you experience these symptoms, reduce the frequency of application, dilute the solution further, or discontinue use.

- **Allergic Reactions:** Although rare, allergic reactions to DMSO are possible. These can manifest as hives, rash, or difficulty breathing. If you suspect an allergic reaction, seek immediate medical attention.
- **Garlic-like Odor:** DMSO can cause a temporary garlic-like odor on the breath and skin. This is a normal side effect and usually subsides within a few hours.
- **Other Systemic Effects:** In some cases, topical DMSO application can lead to systemic effects, such as headache, nausea, or dizziness. If you experience these symptoms, discontinue use and consult your healthcare provider.

## 7. Important Considerations

- **Drug Interactions:** DMSO can interact with certain medications, increasing their absorption or altering their effects. Always inform your healthcare provider about all medications you are taking, including over-the-counter drugs and supplements, before using DMSO.
- **Medical Conditions:** If you have any underlying health conditions, such as liver or kidney disease, consult your healthcare provider before using DMSO.
- **Pregnancy and Breastfeeding:** The safety of DMSO use during pregnancy and breastfeeding has not been established. It's best to avoid using DMSO during these times unless specifically advised by your healthcare provider.

## 8. Seeking Professional Guidance

- **Consult Your Doctor:** Always consult your healthcare provider before using DMSO for any health condition, especially if you are pregnant, breastfeeding, have any underlying health conditions, or are taking any medications.

- **Reliable Sources:** Seek information about DMSO from reputable sources, such as medical journals, healthcare professionals, and trusted websites. Avoid relying solely on anecdotal evidence or unverified claims.

## Can DMSO be Used with Other Skin Treatments or Medications

Combining DMSO with other skin treatments or medications is a topic that requires careful consideration and professional guidance. While DMSO has the remarkable ability to enhance the absorption of other substances through the skin, this very property can also lead to unintended consequences and potential risks if not approached cautiously.

Here's a comprehensive exploration of the factors to consider when using DMSO with other skin treatments:

### Understanding the Risks and Benefits

DMSO's role as a "carrier" molecule means it can significantly increase the penetration of other substances into your bloodstream. This can be beneficial in some cases, such as when using DMSO to improve the delivery of certain medications. However, it also means that any side effects or risks associated with those substances can be amplified.

### Factors to Consider

- **The Specific Skin Treatment or Medication:** The nature of the other treatment or medication you're considering using with DMSO is paramount. Some substances are known to interact with DMSO in potentially harmful ways, while others may be safe or even have synergistic effects. It's crucial to research the specific substance in question and consult with your healthcare provider to assess the potential risks and benefits.

- **Concentration and Dilution:** The concentration of both DMSO and the other substance plays a significant role in determining the overall effect. Higher concentrations can lead to increased absorption and potentially more pronounced side effects. Proper dilution is often necessary to ensure safety and effectiveness. Always follow recommended dilution guidelines or consult with a healthcare professional.

- **Application Method:** The way you apply DMSO and the other substance can also influence their interaction. For example, applying them simultaneously versus sequentially can affect absorption rates and potential interactions. Consider the specific instructions for each substance and consult with your healthcare provider for guidance on the best application method.

- **Individual Factors:** Your individual health status, skin sensitivity, and any existing medical conditions can also influence how your skin reacts to the combination of DMSO and other treatments. If you have sensitive skin or any known allergies, it's essential to proceed with caution and consult with your healthcare provider before trying any new combinations.

**Potential Interactions and Risks**

- **Increased Side Effects:** As mentioned earlier, DMSO can amplify the side effects of other substances. This means that if a particular medication has potential side effects like skin irritation, redness, or itching, using it with DMSO could make these side effects more pronounced.

- **Unpredictable Reactions:** Combining DMSO with certain substances can lead to unpredictable chemical reactions or byproducts. These reactions could potentially cause skin irritation, allergic reactions, or other adverse effects.

- **Systemic Absorption:** DMSO can facilitate the absorption of substances into your bloodstream, which can be beneficial for certain medications. However, it also means that substances not intended for systemic absorption could enter your bloodstream and potentially cause unintended effects.

- **Drug Interactions:** DMSO can interact with certain medications you may be taking orally or through other routes. These interactions could alter the effectiveness of the medications or increase the risk of side effects. Always inform your healthcare provider about all medications you're taking, including any topical treatments, before using DMSO.

**Examples of Specific Interactions**

- **Corticosteroids:** DMSO can enhance the absorption of topical corticosteroids, which can be helpful in treating certain skin conditions. However, it can also increase the risk of side effects like skin thinning and adrenal suppression.

- **Anti-inflammatory Drugs:** DMSO may increase the absorption of certain anti-inflammatory drugs, potentially leading to increased effectiveness but also a higher risk of side effects.

- **Chemotherapy Drugs:** There's some evidence that DMSO can interfere with the effectiveness of certain chemotherapy drugs. If you're undergoing cancer treatment, it's crucial to avoid using DMSO without consulting your oncologist.

- **Blood Thinners:** DMSO may increase the effects of blood thinners, potentially increasing the risk of bleeding.
- **Heart Medications:** DMSO can interact with certain heart medications, potentially altering their effectiveness or increasing the risk of side effects.

**Recommendations and Precautions**

- **Consult Your Healthcare Provider:** The most important recommendation is to always consult with your healthcare provider before using DMSO with any other skin treatment or medication. They can assess your individual situation, consider potential risks and benefits, and provide personalized guidance.
- **Start with a Small Test Area:** If you're considering combining DMSO with another treatment, start by applying it to a small, inconspicuous area of skin to observe for any adverse reactions.
- **Monitor for Side Effects:** Pay close attention to any changes in your skin or overall health after using DMSO with other treatments. If you notice any unusual symptoms, discontinue use and contact your healthcare provider.
- **Follow Instructions Carefully:** Always follow the instructions provided for both DMSO and the other treatment or medication. Pay attention to concentration, dilution, and application methods.
- **Use Pharmaceutical-Grade DMSO:** Ensure you're using pharmaceutical-grade DMSO to minimize the risk of contaminants that could interact with other treatments.

- **Keep a Record:** Keep a record of the treatments you're using, including concentrations, dilutions, and application methods. This information can be helpful for your healthcare provider in assessing any potential interactions or side effects.

By approaching the combination of DMSO with other skin treatments or medications with caution and seeking professional guidance, you can minimize potential risks and maximize the chances of achieving safe and effective outcomes.

# CHAPTER SIX
## **DMSO and Other Ailments**

While DMSO has garnered significant attention for its potential therapeutic applications, it's crucial to remember that its official approval from the U.S. Food and Drug Administration (FDA) is limited to a single use: the treatment of interstitial cystitis, a painful bladder condition.

Despite this limited approval, DMSO has a rich history of being used for a wide range of other health conditions, often referred to as "off-label" uses. These uses haven't undergone the rigorous testing and scrutiny required for FDA approval, meaning their safety and effectiveness aren't fully established.

It's important to approach these off-label uses with a balanced perspective, considering both the anecdotal evidence and the potential risks. Always consult with your healthcare provider before using DMSO for any health concern, especially if you have pre-existing conditions or are taking other medications.

Here's a closer look at some of the health problems for which people have turned to DMSO, even without official approval:

**1. Musculoskeletal Conditions**

- **Arthritis:** DMSO's anti-inflammatory properties have led many people to use it topically for various forms of arthritis, including osteoarthritis and rheumatoid arthritis. Some believe it can help reduce pain, swelling, and stiffness in affected joints.

- **Muscle Injuries:** Athletes and those with muscle strains, sprains, or other injuries sometimes apply DMSO to promote healing and reduce pain.

The idea is that DMSO's ability to penetrate tissues might help deliver its anti-inflammatory effects directly to the injured area.

- **Tendonitis and Bursitis:** These conditions involve inflammation of the tendons and bursae (fluid-filled sacs that cushion joints). DMSO is sometimes used in an attempt to reduce inflammation and alleviate pain.

- **Back Pain:** DMSO may be applied topically to the lower back in an effort to relieve pain associated with conditions like sciatica or muscle spasms.

## 2. Skin Conditions

- **Wound Healing:** DMSO is believed to promote wound healing by increasing blood flow to the affected area, reducing inflammation, and potentially stimulating cell growth. Some people use it for minor cuts, scrapes, and burns.

- **Scars:** There's anecdotal evidence suggesting that DMSO might help reduce the appearance of scars, possibly by softening scar tissue and improving collagen production.

- **Skin Infections:** Some proponents believe DMSO's antimicrobial properties could help with certain skin infections, though this hasn't been scientifically proven.

- **Shingles:** Though not FDA-approved for this use, some healthcare providers use DMSO to manage the pain associated with shingles, a viral infection that causes a painful rash.

## 3. Neurological Conditions

- **Headaches:** Some individuals report finding relief from headaches, including migraines, by applying DMSO topically to the temples or forehead.

- **Stroke:** While research is limited and inconclusive, there's some interest in exploring DMSO's potential to reduce damage after a stroke. This is based on its ability to reduce inflammation and potentially protect nerve cells.

- **Spinal Cord Injuries:** Similar to stroke, there's early research investigating whether DMSO might have a role in minimizing damage and promoting recovery after spinal cord injuries.

## 4. Other Conditions

- **Respiratory Problems:** DMSO has been used in some cases to try to alleviate symptoms of respiratory conditions like asthma and bronchitis. It's thought that its anti-inflammatory effects might help reduce airway inflammation.

- **Eye Problems:** Although controversial, some alternative medicine practitioners use DMSO eye drops for conditions like cataracts and glaucoma. However, this use carries significant risks and is generally discouraged by mainstream ophthalmologists.

- **Cancer:** The use of DMSO for cancer is highly controversial. While some proponents claim it can shrink tumors or enhance the effects of chemotherapy, there's no strong scientific evidence to support these claims. Using DMSO for cancer could delay or interfere with conventional cancer treatments, which is why it's crucial to consult with an oncologist before considering it.

- **Autoimmune Diseases:** Due to its anti-inflammatory effects, DMSO has been explored as a potential treatment for autoimmune conditions like lupus and scleroderma. However, more research is needed to determine its safety and effectiveness in these cases.

- **Mental Health Conditions:** There's very limited and preliminary research looking at DMSO's potential effects on mental health conditions like depression and anxiety. However, these are early explorations, and much more research is needed.

## **DMSO's Mechanisms of Action**

DMSO is not FDA-approved for the treatment of many conditions, anecdotal evidence and preliminary research suggest it may have potential benefits for a variety of ailments. It's crucial to emphasize that these potential benefits are often based on limited studies and anecdotal reports, and further research is necessary to confirm its efficacy and safety for these uses. However, understanding how DMSO works can provide insights into why people use it for these conditions. DMSO exhibits several properties that may contribute to its potential therapeutic effects:

- **Anti-inflammatory:** DMSO is believed to reduce inflammation by inhibiting the production of inflammatory chemicals in the body. This anti-inflammatory action may be responsible for its reported pain-relieving effects in conditions like arthritis, muscle injuries, and nerve pain.

- **Antioxidant:** DMSO acts as a scavenger of free radicals, unstable molecules that can damage cells and contribute to various diseases. By neutralizing these free radicals, DMSO may help protect cells from oxidative stress and reduce the risk of chronic conditions.

- **Analgesic (Pain Relief):** DMSO may block nerve conduction fibers that produce pain, leading to a reduction in pain perception. This analgesic effect may be particularly useful in conditions like neuropathic pain, where conventional pain medications are often ineffective.

- **Vasodilation:** DMSO can cause blood vessels to dilate, increasing blood flow to the affected area. This improved circulation may promote healing and reduce inflammation.

- **Enhanced Drug Absorption:** DMSO's ability to penetrate the skin and other biological membranes makes it a useful carrier for other medications. It can help transport drugs across the skin barrier, potentially increasing their effectiveness and reducing the need for higher doses.

- **Muscle Relaxant:** DMSO may help relax muscles and reduce muscle spasms, which can be beneficial in conditions like muscle strains, sprains, and back pain.

- **Diuretic:** DMSO may increase urine production, which can be helpful in conditions where fluid retention is a problem.

## Potential Applications in Specific Conditions

Based on these mechanisms of action, here's how DMSO might potentially help with various ailments, even though it's not FDA-approved for these uses:

- **Arthritis:** DMSO's anti-inflammatory and analgesic properties may help reduce pain and stiffness associated with arthritis. Some people apply it topically to affected joints, while others report benefits from oral or intravenous administration.

- **Muscle Injuries:** DMSO may help reduce pain, inflammation, and muscle spasms associated with muscle strains, sprains, and tears. Its ability to enhance drug absorption may also make it useful for delivering other pain medications or anti-inflammatory agents to the injured area.

- **Nerve Pain (Neuropathy):** DMSO's analgesic and anti-inflammatory effects may help relieve nerve pain, including conditions like diabetic neuropathy, post-herpetic neuralgia, and complex regional pain syndrome.

- **Headaches:** Some people report that applying DMSO topically to the temples or forehead can help relieve headaches, possibly due to its analgesic and muscle relaxant properties.

- **Respiratory Problems:** DMSO has been used in some cases to help alleviate symptoms of respiratory conditions like bronchitis and asthma. Its anti-inflammatory effects may help reduce airway inflammation, while its ability to break up mucus may help clear congestion.

- **Skin Conditions:** DMSO's anti-inflammatory and antioxidant properties may be beneficial for various skin conditions, including:
    - **Wound Healing:** DMSO may promote wound healing by increasing blood flow to the area, reducing inflammation, and protecting cells from damage.
    - **Burns:** DMSO may help reduce pain, inflammation, and scarring associated with burns.
    - **Scars:** Some people use DMSO to reduce the appearance of scars, although its effectiveness for this purpose is not well-established.

- **Skin Infections:** DMSO's ability to penetrate the skin may make it useful for delivering antifungal or antibacterial medications to treat skin infections.

- **Cancer:** It's crucial to approach this topic with extreme caution. While some preliminary research suggests that DMSO may have anti-cancer properties, there is no conclusive evidence to support its use as a cancer treatment. The use of DMSO for cancer should only be considered under the strict guidance of a qualified healthcare professional.

- **Other Conditions:** DMSO has been explored for its potential benefits in a wide range of other conditions, including:
  - **Interstitial Cystitis:** This is the only condition for which DMSO is FDA-approved. It's administered directly into the bladder to reduce pain and inflammation.
  - **Amyloidosis:** DMSO may help break down amyloid deposits, abnormal protein accumulations that can cause organ damage.
  - **Scleroderma:** DMSO may help soften and improve the flexibility of skin affected by scleroderma, a condition that causes hardening and tightening of the skin.
  - **Gastrointestinal Problems:** DMSO may help reduce inflammation in the digestive tract and alleviate symptoms of conditions like irritable bowel syndrome (IBS) and Crohn's disease.

DMSO has shown promise in some areas and has been used anecdotally for various conditions, it's crucial to approach its use for serious conditions like cancer with extreme caution and a healthy dose of skepticism. Here's why:

## 1. Lack of Robust Scientific Evidence

- **Limited Clinical Trials:** While some laboratory studies have suggested that DMSO might have anti-cancer properties (e.g., inducing cell differentiation, inhibiting tumor growth), these findings haven't been consistently replicated in large-scale, well-controlled clinical trials on humans.

- **No FDA Approval for Cancer Treatment:** The FDA has not approved DMSO for any type of cancer treatment. This means it hasn't undergone the rigorous testing required to demonstrate its safety and effectiveness for this purpose.

- **Anecdotal Evidence is Not Enough:** While there may be anecdotal reports or testimonials from individuals who believe DMSO helped them with cancer, these accounts are not a substitute for scientific evidence. Anecdotes can be biased, influenced by other factors, and don't provide the controlled data needed to draw reliable conclusions.

## 2. Potential Risks and Complications

- **Unknown Long-Term Effects:** The long-term effects of using DMSO, especially in high doses or for extended periods, are not well-understood. This is particularly concerning for cancer patients who may already be dealing with compromised health.

- **Drug Interactions:** DMSO can interact with various medications, including chemotherapy drugs.

- These interactions could reduce the effectiveness of conventional treatments or increase the risk of side effects.
- **Side Effects:** While generally considered safe when used correctly, DMSO can cause side effects, including skin irritation, allergic reactions, a garlic-like taste in the mouth and body odor. In some cases, it can cause more serious issues like headaches, dizziness, and nausea. These side effects can be particularly challenging for cancer patients already experiencing treatment-related side effects.
- **Delaying or Interfering with Proven Treatments:** Perhaps the most significant risk of using DMSO for cancer is that it might lead people to delay or forgo conventional cancer treatments that have a proven track record. This could have serious consequences for their health and prognosis.

## 3. The Complexity of Cancer

- **Cancer is Not a Single Disease:** Cancer is a complex group of diseases with different types, stages, and characteristics. What might work for one type of cancer may not work for another. There's no guarantee that DMSO will be effective for any specific cancer.
- **Individualized Treatment:** Cancer treatment is increasingly personalized, taking into account the individual's specific cancer type, genetic makeup, and overall health. Using DMSO without a proper medical evaluation and integration into a comprehensive treatment plan could be counterproductive.

## 4. Ethical Concerns

- **Exploiting Hope:** Cancer patients are often vulnerable and desperate for solutions. Promoting DMSO as a cancer treatment without strong scientific backing can exploit this hope and lead to false expectations.

- **Financial Exploitation:** Some unscrupulous individuals or companies might promote and sell DMSO products for cancer at exorbitant prices, taking advantage of people's desperation.

## 5. The Importance of Medical Supervision

- **Informed Decision-Making:** If someone is considering using DMSO for cancer, it's crucial to have a thorough discussion with their oncologist or other qualified healthcare professional. This discussion should include:
    - The potential benefits and risks of DMSO
    - The available scientific evidence (or lack thereof)
    - How DMSO might interact with their current cancer treatment
    - The potential for DMSO to interfere with or delay conventional treatment

- **Integrated Approach:** If DMSO is to be used, it should be part of an integrated treatment plan developed in consultation with a healthcare professional. It should not be seen as a replacement for proven cancer therapies.

While DMSO may have potential applications in some areas of medicine, its use for serious conditions like cancer should be approached with extreme caution.

The lack of strong scientific evidence, potential risks, and ethical concerns necessitate a careful and informed decision-making process. Always consult with a qualified healthcare professional before considering DMSO for cancer or any other serious health condition. Never let hope overshadow sound medical judgment and the importance of evidence-based treatment.

# CHAPTER SEVEN
## **DMSO and Animals**

DMSO, with its unique ability to penetrate tissues and carry other substances along with it, has found a place in veterinary medicine for a variety of applications. While its use in animals is often considered "off-label" (meaning not specifically approved by regulatory agencies for those species), veterinarians utilize its properties to address a range of conditions in horses, dogs, and even other animals.

### **DMSO in Horses**

In the equine world, DMSO has gained a reputation for its versatility in managing various health issues.

- **Musculoskeletal Problems:** One of the most common uses of DMSO in horses is for musculoskeletal problems. Its anti-inflammatory properties can help reduce swelling and pain associated with sprains, strains, tendonitis, and arthritis. DMSO is often applied topically to the affected area, either as a solution or gel. It can also be administered intravenously in cases of severe inflammation or when a systemic effect is desired.

- **Laminitis:** Laminitis, a painful and potentially debilitating condition affecting the hooves, is another area where DMSO is often employed. Its ability to reduce inflammation and improve blood flow can be beneficial in managing the acute phase of laminitis. DMSO is typically given intravenously in these cases, often in conjunction with other therapies.

- **Wound Healing:** DMSO's ability to penetrate tissues and reduce inflammation can also be helpful in wound healing. It can be applied topically to wounds to promote healing and reduce scarring.

However, it's important to use caution with open wounds, as DMSO can carry contaminants into the wound if it's not pure.

- **Neurological Conditions:** In some cases, DMSO has been used in horses with neurological conditions, such as spinal cord injuries or brain swelling. Its potential to reduce inflammation and oxidative stress may play a role in these applications, although more research is needed in this area.

## <u>DMSO in Dogs</u>

While DMSO is used less extensively in dogs compared to horses, it still has some valuable applications.

- **Skin Conditions:** Topical DMSO can be helpful in managing certain skin conditions in dogs, such as lick granulomas (acral lick dermatitis) and calcinosis cutis (calcium deposits in the skin). Its anti-inflammatory effects and ability to enhance the penetration of other topical medications can be beneficial in these cases.

- **Bladder Conditions:** DMSO is sometimes used in the treatment of hemorrhagic cystitis (inflammation of the bladder with bleeding) in dogs. It can be instilled directly into the bladder to reduce inflammation and pain.

- **Ear Infections:** In some cases, DMSO may be used as an ear drop for certain types of ear infections in dogs. Its anti-inflammatory and antimicrobial properties may contribute to its effectiveness.

## <u>DMSO in Other Animals</u>

While horses and dogs are the most common recipients of DMSO therapy, it has also been used in other animal species, including:

- **Cats:** Similar to dogs, DMSO may be used topically for skin conditions or instilled into the bladder for cystitis in cats.

- **Cattle:** DMSO has been used in cattle for various purposes, including the treatment of mastitis (inflammation of the udder) and ketosis (a metabolic disorder).
- **Exotic Animals:** In some cases, DMSO may be used in exotic animals, such as birds and reptiles, for specific conditions under the guidance of a veterinarian experienced in these species.

## Important Considerations for Animal Use

- **Veterinary Supervision:** It's crucial to emphasize that DMSO should only be used in animals under the guidance and supervision of a veterinarian. They can properly assess the animal's condition, determine the appropriate dosage and route of administration, and monitor for any potential side effects.
- **Purity and Quality:** Just as with human use, it's essential to use only pharmaceutical-grade DMSO for animals. Impurities in lower-grade DMSO can be harmful to animals.
- **Species-Specific Considerations:** Different animal species may metabolize and respond to DMSO differently. Veterinarians take these factors into account when determining the appropriate use and dosage.
- **Potential Side Effects:** DMSO can cause side effects in animals, including skin irritation, gastrointestinal upset, and changes in blood parameters. Monitoring for these effects is important.
- **Withdrawal Times:** For animals used for food production, such as cattle, there are withdrawal times associated with DMSO use. This means that a certain amount of time must pass after the last DMSO administration before the animal's milk or meat can be safely consumed by humans.

While DMSO has been used in veterinary medicine for several decades, research continues to explore its potential applications and optimize its use in various species. As our understanding of DMSO's mechanisms and effects grows, it's likely that its role in animal health will continue to evolve.

By using DMSO responsibly and under the guidance of a veterinarian, we can harness its unique properties to improve the health and well-being of our animal companions.

## Safety Considerations in Using DMSO to Treat Animals

DMSO has shown promise in veterinary medicine for various applications, it's crucial to approach its use with caution and a thorough understanding of its potential effects on animals. Just as with humans, responsible use involves careful consideration of the animal's health, the specific condition being treated, and adherence to proper administration techniques.

Here's a comprehensive look at the safety considerations when using DMSO for animals:

### 1. Species-Specific Sensitivities

- **Varied Responses:** Different animal species can react to DMSO in unique ways. What might be safe for a horse might not be suitable for a cat or a dog. It's essential to research and understand the specific sensitivities of the animal you're treating.

- **Cats and DMSO:** For instance, cats are known to be more sensitive to DMSO than some other species. They may experience more pronounced side effects, such as red blood cell damage, if DMSO is administered incorrectly or in high doses.

This sensitivity underscores the importance of consulting a veterinarian experienced in DMSO therapy for cats.

## 2. Underlying Health Conditions

- **Pre-existing Conditions:** An animal's overall health and any underlying medical conditions can influence how they tolerate DMSO. Liver or kidney problems, for example, may necessitate lower doses or a different treatment approach altogether.

- **Medication Interactions:** Just as with humans, DMSO can interact with certain medications. If the animal is on any other medications, it's crucial to discuss potential interactions with your veterinarian before starting DMSO therapy.

## 3. Administration Route and Dosage

- **Multiple Routes:** DMSO can be administered to animals through various routes, including topical, intravenous, and oral. The choice of route depends on the condition being treated and the animal's individual needs.

- **Topical Application:** For topical use, it's important to clean the area thoroughly before applying DMSO. The concentration of DMSO should be adjusted based on the animal's size and the severity of the condition.

- **Intravenous Administration:** Intravenous DMSO should only be administered by a qualified veterinarian. Careful monitoring is necessary to avoid potential complications.

- **Oral Administration:** Oral DMSO can cause a garlic-like taste in the mouth and may lead to bad breath. Some animals may be reluctant to take it orally.

- **Dosage Accuracy:** Accurate dosing is critical. Overdosing can increase the risk of side effects, while underdosing may render the treatment ineffective. Always follow your veterinarian's dosage recommendations carefully.

## 4. Potential Side Effects

- **Common Side Effects:** Some common side effects of DMSO in animals include skin irritation, redness, dryness, or a garlic-like odor on the animal's breath and skin. These effects are usually mild and temporary.

- **Serious Side Effects:** In some cases, more serious side effects can occur, such as:
  - **Gastrointestinal Upset:** Nausea, vomiting, or diarrhea may occur, especially with oral administration.
  - **Allergic Reactions:** Although rare, allergic reactions can happen. Watch for signs like hives, facial swelling, or difficulty breathing. If you suspect an allergic reaction, seek immediate veterinary attention.
  - **Central Nervous System Effects:** In rare instances, DMSO can cause central nervous system effects like drowsiness, dizziness, or seizures.
  - **Blood Abnormalities:** As mentioned earlier, cats may be more prone to red blood cell damage with DMSO use.

## 5. Monitoring and Follow-Up

- **Observation:** After administering DMSO, closely monitor the animal for any adverse reactions or changes in behavior. If you notice anything unusual, contact your veterinarian.

- **Follow-Up Care:** Regular check-ups with your veterinarian are essential to assess the effectiveness of the treatment and make any necessary adjustments to the dosage or administration route.

## 6. Special Considerations

- **Pregnant or Nursing Animals:** The safety of DMSO in pregnant or nursing animals has not been fully established. It's best to avoid using it in these situations unless specifically directed by your veterinarian.

- **Young Animals:** Young animals may be more susceptible to the effects of DMSO. Use with caution and under the guidance of a veterinarian.

- **Competition Animals:** Regulations regarding DMSO use in competition animals vary. Check with the relevant governing bodies to ensure compliance.

## 7. Choosing a Veterinarian

- **Experience with DMSO:** Not all veterinarians have experience with DMSO therapy. Seek out a veterinarian who is knowledgeable about DMSO and its use in animals. They can provide tailored advice and guidance based on your animal's specific needs.

By taking these safety considerations seriously and working closely with your veterinarian, you can help ensure that DMSO therapy is as safe and effective as possible for your animal companion. Remember, responsible use is key to maximizing the potential benefits of DMSO while minimizing any risks.

# Part 3: Maximizing DMSO's Potential

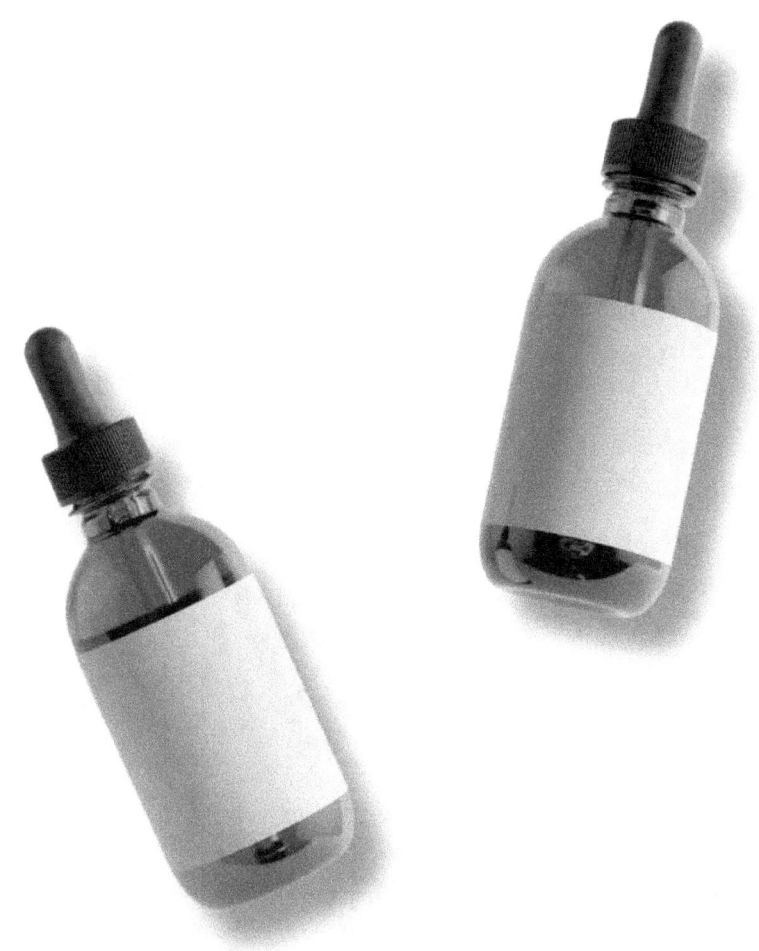

# CHAPTER EIGHT
## Combining DMSO with Other Therapies

DMSO can often be used alongside other treatments and therapies, and in some cases, this combination may even enhance its potential benefits. However, it's crucial to approach this with caution and awareness, as DMSO's interactions with other substances can be complex and sometimes unpredictable. Here's a deeper dive into how DMSO can be integrated with other therapies:

DMSO's unique properties make it a potentially valuable adjunct to various treatments. Its ability to penetrate the skin and biological membranes allows it to act as a carrier, enhancing the absorption of other substances. This can be particularly beneficial for topical medications or natural remedies, increasing their effectiveness and potentially reducing the required dosage. Additionally, DMSO's anti-inflammatory and antioxidant properties may complement other therapies aimed at reducing pain, inflammation, or oxidative stress.

### Combining DMSO with Conventional Medical Treatments

- **Topical Medications:** DMSO can be used in conjunction with certain topical medications to improve their penetration and efficacy. For instance, it may be used with antifungal creams for skin infections, or with pain-relieving gels for arthritis. However, it's essential to consult with your doctor before combining DMSO with any prescription medication, as there could be potential interactions or contraindications.

- **Injectable Medications:** In some cases, DMSO is used as a solvent for injectable medications, aiding in their delivery and distribution within the body. This is often done under strict medical supervision.

- **Physical Therapy:** DMSO may be used as part of a comprehensive physical therapy program for musculoskeletal injuries or pain conditions. Its anti-inflammatory effects can help reduce pain and swelling, allowing for more effective physical therapy sessions.

## Integrating DMSO with Complementary and Alternative Therapies

- **Essential Oils:** DMSO can be used as a carrier for essential oils, enhancing their absorption through the skin. This can be particularly useful for aromatherapy or topical applications of essential oils for pain relief, relaxation, or skin conditions. However, it's important to choose high-quality essential oils and dilute them appropriately before use.

- **Herbal Remedies:** Similar to essential oils, DMSO can improve the absorption of herbal extracts or tinctures applied topically. This can potentially increase their therapeutic effects.

- **Nutritional Supplements:** While there's limited research in this area, some practitioners suggest that DMSO may enhance the absorption of certain nutritional supplements, particularly those applied topically.

- **Acupuncture and Massage:** Some practitioners use DMSO in conjunction with acupuncture or massage therapy. The theory is that DMSO's anti-inflammatory and pain-relieving properties may complement these therapies, promoting relaxation and reducing muscle tension.

# **Specific Combined Therapies**

## **DMSO and Magnesium Chloride for Muscle Pain**

When it comes to muscle pain, many people seek relief beyond conventional treatments. This is where the combination of DMSO and magnesium chloride enters the picture, offering a potential natural approach to managing discomfort. Let's delve into the fascinating world of these two substances and how they might work together to alleviate muscle pain.

Dimethyl sulfoxide (DMSO) is a colorless, slightly oily liquid derived from wood pulp. It's known for its remarkable ability to penetrate the skin and other biological membranes, carrying other substances along with it. This unique characteristic makes DMSO a valuable tool in various applications, from industrial uses to potential therapeutic benefits.

While DMSO is officially approved by the FDA only for the treatment of interstitial cystitis (a painful bladder condition), its potential benefits for muscle pain have garnered significant interest. Although research in this area is still ongoing and more studies are needed to confirm its efficacy, anecdotal evidence and preliminary findings suggest that DMSO may offer several mechanisms for muscle pain relief:

- **Reducing Inflammation:** DMSO is believed to possess anti-inflammatory properties, which can help soothe inflamed muscles and reduce pain. It may achieve this by inhibiting the production of inflammatory chemicals in the body.

- **Blocking Pain Signals:** DMSO may interfere with the transmission of pain signals along nerve fibers, leading to a decrease in pain perception.

- **Increasing Blood Flow:** By promoting blood circulation to the affected area, DMSO may help deliver oxygen and nutrients to the muscles, aiding in the healing process.
- **Relaxing Muscles:** Some proponents suggest that DMSO may help relax muscle tension and spasms, further contributing to pain relief.

Magnesium is a vital mineral involved in numerous bodily functions, including muscle contraction and relaxation, nerve transmission, and energy production. Magnesium deficiency can lead to muscle cramps, spasms, and pain.

Magnesium chloride is a highly absorbable form of magnesium that can be applied topically or taken orally. When applied to the skin, magnesium chloride is believed to be absorbed into the muscles, where it can exert its beneficial effects:

- **Restoring Magnesium Levels:** Topical application of magnesium chloride can help replenish magnesium levels in muscle tissues, reducing the likelihood of cramps and spasms.
- **Relaxing Muscle Fibers:** Magnesium plays a crucial role in muscle relaxation by counteracting the effects of calcium, which is involved in muscle contraction.
- **Reducing Inflammation:** Magnesium may also have anti-inflammatory effects, further contributing to pain relief.

The combination of DMSO and magnesium chloride may offer a synergistic effect in managing muscle pain. DMSO's ability to penetrate the skin can enhance the absorption of magnesium chloride into the muscles, allowing it to reach the site of pain more effectively.

This combination is often used topically in the form of creams, gels, or sprays. Anecdotal reports suggest that it may be helpful for various muscle-related issues, including:

- **Muscle Soreness and Stiffness:** Whether from exercise, injury, or chronic conditions like fibromyalgia, the combination may help alleviate pain and improve flexibility.
- **Muscle Cramps and Spasms:** By replenishing magnesium levels and promoting muscle relaxation, this combination may help reduce the frequency and intensity of muscle cramps.
- **Back Pain:** Many individuals find relief from back pain by applying DMSO and magnesium chloride to the affected area.

While the combination of DMSO and magnesium chloride shows promise for muscle pain relief, it's essential to approach its use with caution and awareness:

- **Consult Your Doctor:** Always consult your healthcare provider before using DMSO or magnesium chloride, especially if you have any underlying health conditions, are taking medications, or are pregnant or breastfeeding.
- **Source and Purity:** Use only pharmaceutical-grade DMSO and high-quality magnesium chloride from reputable sources.
- **Skin Sensitivity:** DMSO can sometimes cause skin irritation or allergic reactions. Start with a small test area before applying it to larger areas. Diluting DMSO with water can also help reduce skin sensitivity.

- **Application:** When applying topically, follow recommended guidelines and avoid contact with eyes and mucous membranes.
- **Side Effects:** Be aware of potential side effects, such as skin irritation, garlic-like body odor, and gastrointestinal upset (if magnesium chloride is taken orally).

As research continues to explore the therapeutic potential of DMSO and magnesium chloride, we may gain a better understanding of their effectiveness and safety for muscle pain. While anecdotal evidence and preliminary findings are promising, more rigorous studies are needed to confirm their benefits and establish optimal usage guidelines.

In the meantime, individuals seeking natural approaches to muscle pain management may find the combination of DMSO and magnesium chloride worth exploring under the guidance of their healthcare provider. By staying informed and using these substances responsibly, individuals can make empowered choices about their health and well-being.

## **DMSO and Curcumin for Inflammation**

The combination of DMSO and curcumin presents a fascinating area of exploration in the realm of natural remedies for inflammation. Both substances have long histories of traditional use, and modern science is beginning to shed light on their potential synergistic effects. Let's delve into the intriguing world of DMSO and curcumin for inflammation.

Before we explore their combined potential, it's essential to understand each substance individually.

- **DMSO (Dimethyl Sulfoxide):** As we've discussed, DMSO is a potent solvent derived from wood pulp.

It possesses remarkable transdermal properties, meaning it can easily penetrate the skin and carry other substances along with it. This makes it a valuable vehicle for enhancing the absorption of topical medications. DMSO itself also has anti-inflammatory properties, likely due to its ability to scavenge free radicals, reduce inflammatory cytokines, and alter cell membrane permeability.

- **Curcumin:** This vibrant yellow compound is the primary active ingredient in turmeric, a spice widely used in Indian cuisine and traditional medicine. Curcumin has garnered significant attention for its potent anti-inflammatory and antioxidant effects. It works by inhibiting various molecules involved in the inflammatory process, including NF-κB, COX-2, and LOX.

The combination of DMSO and curcumin offers a compelling strategy for addressing inflammation for several reasons:

- **Enhanced Absorption:** Curcumin's bioavailability (the extent to which it's absorbed and utilized by the body) is relatively low when taken orally. This is where DMSO shines. By acting as a carrier, DMSO can significantly improve the absorption of curcumin through the skin, allowing it to reach deeper tissues and exert its anti-inflammatory effects more effectively.

- **Complementary Mechanisms:** DMSO and curcumin appear to work through different pathways to reduce inflammation. DMSO primarily targets free radicals and cell membrane permeability, while curcumin modulates inflammatory signaling molecules. This multi-pronged approach could potentially provide a more comprehensive anti-inflammatory effect.

- **Reduced Side Effects:** When curcumin is taken orally in high doses, it can sometimes cause gastrointestinal issues like nausea and diarrhea. Topical application with DMSO can help bypass these side effects while still delivering therapeutic benefits.

While research on the specific combination of DMSO and curcumin is still somewhat limited, there's growing evidence to support their individual and potentially synergistic effects in managing inflammation:

- **Preclinical Studies:** Laboratory studies have shown that DMSO can enhance the delivery of curcumin into cells and tissues, increasing its anti-inflammatory potency. For example, a study published in the *Journal of Inflammation* found that a combination of curcuma DMSO extract (an extract of turmeric using DMSO as the solvent) and curcumin reduced levels of various inflammatory markers in human intervertebral disc cells.

- **Anecdotal Evidence:** Many individuals report positive experiences using DMSO and curcumin topically for conditions like arthritis, muscle pain, and skin inflammation. They often describe reduced pain, swelling, and improved mobility.

- **Potential Applications:** Based on the available evidence and anecdotal reports, the combination of DMSO and curcumin holds promise for a range of inflammatory conditions, including:
    - **Musculoskeletal pain:** Arthritis, tendonitis, bursitis, muscle strains
    - **Skin conditions:** Psoriasis, eczema, acne, wound healing

- **Nerve pain:** Neuropathy, sciatica
- **Other inflammatory conditions:** Inflammatory bowel disease, autoimmune diseases

If you're considering using DMSO and curcumin for inflammation, keep these important points in mind:

- **Source and Quality:** Always use pharmaceutical-grade DMSO and high-quality curcumin extract from reputable sources.
- **Preparation:** DMSO and curcumin can be mixed into a topical solution or gel. You can find pre-made formulations or consult a compounding pharmacist to create a customized preparation.
- **Application:** Apply the mixture to the affected area, typically 2-3 times per day. Always perform a patch test first to check for any skin sensitivity.
- **Precautions:** Follow the safety guidelines for handling and storing DMSO as discussed earlier. Be aware that curcumin can stain clothing and skin.
- **Medical Supervision:** Consult your healthcare provider before using DMSO and curcumin, especially if you have any underlying health conditions or are taking medications.

The combination of DMSO and curcumin represents an exciting frontier in natural anti-inflammatory therapies. As research continues to explore their synergistic potential, we can expect to gain a deeper understanding of their mechanisms and optimal applications.

While it's important to acknowledge the current limitations in scientific evidence, the anecdotal reports and preliminary studies offer compelling reasons to be optimistic about the future of DMSO and curcumin in managing inflammation and promoting healing.

## **DMSO and Essential Oils for Respiratory Conditions**

DMSO and essential oils have both garnered attention for their potential benefits in addressing various respiratory conditions. While DMSO is recognized primarily for its anti-inflammatory properties and ability to enhance the absorption of other substances, essential oils offer a wide range of therapeutic effects, including antimicrobial, anti-inflammatory, and decongestant actions.

Combining these two may offer a synergistic approach to respiratory support, though it's crucial to understand the limitations of existing evidence and approach such treatments with caution and informed guidance from a healthcare professional.

DMSO, or dimethyl sulfoxide, is a colorless liquid known for its potent anti-inflammatory effects and its remarkable ability to penetrate the skin and other biological membranes. This unique characteristic makes it a valuable carrier for other substances, enhancing their absorption into the body. While its FDA-approved use is limited to the treatment of interstitial cystitis, DMSO has been explored for its potential benefits in various respiratory conditions.

**Potential Mechanisms of Action in Respiratory Conditions**

- **Reducing Inflammation:** DMSO's primary mechanism of action lies in its anti-inflammatory properties. It is believed to inhibit the production of inflammatory mediators, which are substances that contribute to swelling, pain, and other symptoms associated with respiratory conditions such as bronchitis, asthma, and sinusitis.

- **Enhancing Mucolytic Activity:** DMSO may also help to thin and loosen mucus, making it easier to expel. This can be particularly beneficial in conditions like bronchitis and cystic fibrosis, where thick mucus can obstruct the airways and impair breathing.

- **Improving Drug Delivery:** When combined with other medications, DMSO can facilitate their absorption through the skin or mucous membranes. This can be particularly useful for delivering localized treatment to the respiratory system, potentially reducing systemic side effects.

Essential oils, derived from aromatic plants, have been used for centuries for their therapeutic properties. Many essential oils possess antimicrobial, anti-inflammatory, and decongestant properties, making them potentially valuable tools for managing respiratory conditions.

**Key Essential Oils and Their Potential Benefits**

- **Eucalyptus Oil:** Known for its potent decongestant and expectorant properties, eucalyptus oil can help to open up the airways and loosen mucus. Its main component, cineole, has been shown to possess antiviral and antibacterial properties, making it potentially beneficial in fighting respiratory infections.

- **Peppermint Oil:** With its refreshing and invigorating aroma, peppermint oil contains menthol, a natural decongestant that can help to clear the sinuses and relieve congestion. It also possesses anti-inflammatory and antimicrobial properties.

- **Tea Tree Oil:** Renowned for its broad-spectrum antimicrobial activity, tea tree oil can help to combat various respiratory pathogens, including bacteria and viruses. It may also help to reduce inflammation and soothe irritated airways.

- **Lavender Oil:** Primarily known for its calming and relaxing effects, lavender oil may also help to reduce airway inflammation and promote restful sleep, which is crucial for recovery from respiratory illnesses.

- **Thyme Oil:** Thyme oil is a potent antimicrobial agent that can help to fight respiratory infections. It also possesses expectorant properties, aiding in the removal of mucus from the airways.

The combination of DMSO and essential oils may offer a synergistic approach to respiratory support. DMSO's ability to enhance the absorption of other substances could potentially increase the effectiveness of essential oils when applied topically or through inhalation.

**Possible Applications**

- **Topical Chest Rubs:** Combining DMSO with essential oils like eucalyptus, peppermint, and tea tree oil in a carrier oil (such as coconut oil) can create a chest rub that may help to relieve congestion, reduce inflammation, and fight infection.

- **Inhalation:** Adding a few drops of essential oils like eucalyptus or lavender to a bowl of hot water and inhaling the steam can help to open up the airways and soothe irritated mucous membranes. DMSO could potentially be added to the water as well, though further research is needed to confirm its safety and efficacy in this application.

While the combination of DMSO and essential oils holds promise for respiratory support, it's essential to approach this approach with caution and seek guidance from a qualified healthcare professional.

- **Purity and Quality:** Ensure that both the DMSO and essential oils you use are of high quality and purity. Pharmaceutical-grade DMSO and therapeutic-grade essential oils from reputable sources are recommended.

- **Skin Sensitivity:** DMSO and some essential oils can cause skin irritation or allergic reactions in some individuals. Always perform a patch test before applying to a larger area. Dilute essential oils appropriately in a carrier oil before use.

- **Inhalation Safety:** When inhaling essential oils, use caution and avoid excessive exposure. Pregnant women, young children, and individuals with respiratory conditions should consult with a healthcare professional before using essential oils for inhalation.

- **Drug Interactions:** DMSO can interact with certain medications. Consult with your doctor or pharmacist before using DMSO, especially if you are taking any other medications.

- **Medical Supervision:** It's crucial to seek guidance from a qualified healthcare professional before using DMSO or essential oils for any health condition, especially if you have any underlying health issues or are pregnant or breastfeeding.

While anecdotal evidence suggests that DMSO and essential oils may be beneficial for respiratory conditions, scientific research in this area is limited. More studies are needed to confirm their efficacy and safety, particularly when used in combination.

The combination of DMSO and essential oils presents an intriguing possibility for respiratory support. DMSO's anti-inflammatory properties and its ability to enhance absorption, coupled with the therapeutic effects of essential oils, may offer a synergistic approach to managing respiratory conditions.

However, it's crucial to approach this approach with caution, use high-quality products, and seek guidance from a healthcare professional to ensure safe and effective use.

## **Complementary Therapies that Might Work Well with DMSO**

DMSO has shown promise in various applications, it's important to remember that it's not a magic bullet. Integrating DMSO with complementary therapies can potentially enhance its benefits and address health concerns more holistically. Here are some complementary therapies that might work well in conjunction with DMSO:

### **1. Essential Oils**

Essential oils are concentrated plant extracts that have been used for centuries for their therapeutic properties. Many essential oils possess anti-inflammatory, analgesic, and antimicrobial properties, which can complement DMSO's effects.

- **Synergy with DMSO:** DMSO's ability to penetrate the skin can enhance the absorption and effectiveness of essential oils. When applied topically, DMSO can act as a carrier, helping essential oils reach deeper tissues.

- **Examples:**
    - **Lavender oil:** Known for its calming and relaxing effects, lavender oil can be combined with DMSO for pain relief, anxiety reduction, and improved sleep.

- **Tea tree oil:** This oil has potent antimicrobial properties and can be used with DMSO to treat skin infections, wounds, and burns.
- **Peppermint oil:** With its cooling and analgesic effects, peppermint oil can be added to DMSO for muscle pain, headaches, and joint discomfort.
- **Frankincense oil:** This oil has anti-inflammatory properties and can be combined with DMSO for arthritis, inflammation, and skin conditions.

**Important Considerations:**

- **Quality:** Use high-quality, therapeutic-grade essential oils from reputable sources.
- **Dilution:** Always dilute essential oils properly before applying them topically, especially when combined with DMSO.
- **Sensitivity:** Perform a patch test before applying essential oils to a larger area, as some individuals may be sensitive to certain oils.

## 2. Herbal Remedies

Herbal remedies have been used for centuries in traditional medicine systems to address various health conditions. Many herbs possess anti-inflammatory, antioxidant, and pain-relieving properties, which can complement DMSO's therapeutic effects.

- **Synergy with DMSO:** DMSO can enhance the absorption and delivery of herbal extracts to targeted tissues.

- **Examples:**
  - **Arnica:** This herb is known for its anti-inflammatory and pain-relieving properties and can be used with DMSO for bruises, sprains, and muscle soreness.
  - **Turmeric:** Curcumin, the active compound in turmeric, has potent anti-inflammatory and antioxidant effects. Combining turmeric with DMSO may help with arthritis, joint pain, and skin conditions.
  - **Ginger:** Ginger has anti-inflammatory and analgesic properties and can be used with DMSO for nausea, muscle pain, and headaches.
  - **Aloe vera:** Aloe vera is known for its soothing and healing properties and can be combined with DMSO for burns, wounds, and skin irritations.

**Important Considerations:**

- **Quality:** Choose high-quality herbal products from reputable sources.
- **Interactions:** Be aware of potential interactions between herbs and any medications you may be taking.
- **Consultation:** Consult with a qualified herbalist or healthcare professional before using herbs, especially if you have any underlying health conditions.

### 3. Physical Therapy
Physical therapy involves exercises, stretches, and manual techniques to improve mobility, reduce pain, and restore function. Combining physical therapy with DMSO can potentially enhance the benefits of both approaches.

- **Synergy with DMSO:** DMSO's anti-inflammatory and pain-relieving effects can complement physical therapy by reducing pain and inflammation in muscles and joints, allowing for more effective exercise and rehabilitation.
- **Examples:**
    - **Stretching and range-of-motion exercises:** DMSO can help reduce muscle soreness and stiffness, making stretching and range-of-motion exercises more comfortable and effective.
    - **Strengthening exercises:** DMSO can help reduce pain and inflammation in joints, allowing for more effective strengthening exercises.
    - **Manual therapy:** DMSO can be applied topically before or after manual therapy techniques like massage or joint mobilization to enhance their effects.

**Important Considerations:**

- **Guidance:** Work with a qualified physical therapist to develop a personalized exercise plan.
- **Timing:** Discuss with your physical therapist the optimal timing for applying DMSO in relation to your therapy sessions.

### 4. Mindfulness and Meditation

Mindfulness and meditation practices involve focusing on the present moment and cultivating awareness of thoughts, feelings, and sensations. These practices can help reduce stress, anxiety, and pain perception, which can complement DMSO's therapeutic effects.

- **Synergy with DMSO:** DMSO can help reduce physical discomfort, allowing for more comfortable and focused meditation practice. Mindfulness and meditation can help manage stress and anxiety, which can contribute to pain and inflammation.

- **Examples:**
    - **Mindful breathing:** Practicing mindful breathing exercises can help reduce stress and anxiety, which can complement DMSO's pain-relieving effects.
    - **Body scan meditation:** This practice involves bringing awareness to different parts of the body, which can help identify areas of tension and discomfort. Combining body scan meditation with DMSO application can potentially enhance pain relief.
    - **Guided meditation:** Guided meditations for pain management or relaxation can be used in conjunction with DMSO to promote overall well-being.

**Important Considerations:**

- **Consistency:** Regular practice is key to experiencing the benefits of mindfulness and meditation.
- **Guidance:** Consider seeking guidance from a qualified meditation teacher or therapist.

## 5. Acupuncture

Acupuncture is a traditional Chinese medicine technique that involves inserting thin needles into specific points on the body to stimulate energy flow and promote healing. Acupuncture can be used to address pain, inflammation, and various health conditions.

- **Synergy with DMSO:** DMSO's anti-inflammatory and pain-relieving effects can complement acupuncture's ability to modulate pain signals and reduce inflammation.

- **Examples:**
    - **Pain management:** Acupuncture can be used in conjunction with DMSO to address chronic pain conditions like arthritis, back pain, and headaches.
    - **Inflammation reduction:** Acupuncture can help reduce inflammation throughout the body, complementing DMSO's anti-inflammatory properties.
    - **Stress reduction:** Acupuncture can help reduce stress and anxiety, which can contribute to pain and inflammation.

**Important Considerations:**

- **Qualified Practitioner:** Seek treatment from a licensed and qualified acupuncturist.

- **Combined Approach:** Discuss with your acupuncturist the possibility of combining acupuncture with DMSO and how to optimize the timing and application.

By integrating DMSO with these complementary therapies, you can potentially enhance its benefits and address health concerns in a more holistic and comprehensive way. Remember to consult with your healthcare professional before starting any new therapy or combining it with DMSO to ensure safety and effectiveness.

# CHAPTER NINE
## **DMSO and Lifestyle**

DMSO has shown promise in various applications, it's important to remember that it's not a magic bullet. Its effectiveness can be significantly influenced by your overall lifestyle, including your diet, exercise habits, and stress management techniques. These factors play a crucial role in your body's natural healing and regenerative processes, and they can either amplify or hinder the potential benefits of DMSO.

### Diet:
The food you consume provides the building blocks for your body's cells and tissues, fuels your energy production, and supports countless biochemical reactions. A balanced and nutritious diet can create a favorable environment for healing and regeneration, making your body more receptive to the potential benefits of DMSO.

- **Anti-inflammatory Foods:** DMSO is often used for its anti-inflammatory properties, and you can further enhance these effects by incorporating anti-inflammatory foods into your diet. These include:
    - **Colorful fruits and vegetables:** Berries, leafy greens, tomatoes, and citrus fruits are rich in antioxidants that combat inflammation.
    - **Fatty fish:** Salmon, tuna, and mackerel are excellent sources of omega-3 fatty acids, which have potent anti-inflammatory effects.
    - **Nuts and seeds:** Walnuts, almonds, and flaxseeds provide healthy fats and other nutrients that help reduce inflammation.

- o **Whole grains:** Oats, quinoa, and brown rice offer fiber and other compounds that support a healthy inflammatory response.

- **Hydration:** Staying well-hydrated is crucial for overall health and can also enhance the effectiveness of DMSO. Water helps transport nutrients, flush out toxins, and maintain proper cellular function. Aim to drink plenty of water throughout the day, especially if you're using DMSO topically, as it can have a dehydrating effect on the skin.

- **Limiting Processed Foods:** Processed foods often contain high amounts of sugar, unhealthy fats, and artificial additives that can contribute to inflammation and hinder the body's natural healing processes. By minimizing your intake of these foods, you can create a more supportive environment for DMSO to work its potential benefits.

## Exercise:

Regular physical activity is essential for maintaining optimal health and can also enhance the effects of DMSO. Exercise improves blood circulation, which helps deliver nutrients and oxygen to tissues while removing waste products. This enhanced circulation can facilitate the transport of DMSO to the areas where it's needed most.

- **Types of Exercise:** A well-rounded exercise routine that includes cardiovascular activity, strength training, and flexibility exercises is ideal.
    - o Cardiovascular exercise, such as brisk walking, jogging, or swimming, improves heart health and overall circulation.

- Strength training helps build muscle mass and bone density, which can be particularly beneficial if you're using DMSO for musculoskeletal issues.
- Flexibility exercises, like yoga or stretching, improve range of motion and can help prevent injuries.

- **Tailoring Exercise to Your Needs:** If you're using DMSO for a specific condition, consider incorporating exercises that target that area. For example, if you're using DMSO for knee pain, gentle range-of-motion exercises and low-impact activities like swimming or cycling might be helpful.
- **Listen to Your Body:** It's important to listen to your body and not overdo it, especially if you're dealing with pain or inflammation. Start slowly and gradually increase the intensity and duration of your exercise routine as your body adapts.

## Stress Management:

Chronic stress can take a toll on your physical and mental health, contributing to inflammation, pain, and impaired healing. Effective stress management techniques can help create a more balanced internal environment, allowing your body to better utilize the potential benefits of DMSO.

- **Mindfulness and Relaxation Techniques:** Practices like meditation, deep breathing exercises, and yoga can help calm the nervous system and reduce stress hormones. These techniques can be particularly helpful if you're using DMSO for conditions exacerbated by stress, such as headaches or muscle tension.

- **Adequate Sleep:** Sleep is essential for the body to repair and rejuvenate itself. Aim for 7-9 hours of quality sleep each night to support your overall health and enhance the potential benefits of DMSO.

- **Social Connection:** Strong social connections and a sense of community can provide emotional support and buffer the negative effects of stress. Spending time with loved ones, engaging in hobbies, or participating in group activities can contribute to your overall well-being.

By adopting a holistic approach that includes a healthy diet, regular exercise, and effective stress management, you can create a synergistic effect that amplifies the potential benefits of DMSO. These lifestyle factors work together to support your body's natural healing mechanisms, optimize your overall health, and create a more receptive environment for DMSO to exert its effects.

Remember, DMSO is not a substitute for a healthy lifestyle. It's a tool that can potentially complement your efforts to improve your well-being. By prioritizing your overall health and adopting positive lifestyle habits, you can maximize the potential benefits of DMSO and support your body's innate capacity for healing and regeneration.

# CHAPTER TEN
## **Conclusion**

DMSO, with its remarkable ability to traverse the barriers of our cells, holds a unique place in the landscape of both conventional and alternative medicine. While its FDA-approved use remains limited to the treatment of interstitial cystitis, its potential applications extend far beyond this singular domain. We've seen how DMSO has been explored for its role in alleviating pain and inflammation, promoting wound healing, and even as an adjunct in addressing various skin conditions.

However, it's precisely this versatility that necessitates a cautious and informed approach. DMSO is not a panacea, and it's not without its risks. Its ability to readily penetrate the skin and carry other substances along with it underscores the importance of using only pharmaceutical-grade DMSO and exercising prudence in its application.

Throughout this book, we've emphasized the critical role of collaboration with your healthcare provider. Any decision to incorporate DMSO into your health regimen should be made in consultation with a qualified medical professional. They can assess your individual needs, consider potential interactions with other medications or conditions, and guide you on safe and appropriate usage.

The information presented here is intended for educational purposes and should not be construed as medical advice. It's essential to conduct your own research, consult reliable sources, and remain an active participant in your healthcare decisions.

While DMSO may offer a valuable tool in your health toolkit, it's crucial to recognize that true well-being extends beyond any single remedy. Cultivating a holistic approach to health, encompassing lifestyle factors such as nutrition, exercise, stress management, and emotional well-being, is paramount.

Consider DMSO as a potential adjunct to a foundation of healthy habits. Nourishing your body with wholesome foods, engaging in regular physical activity, prioritizing quality sleep, and cultivating emotional resilience can create a fertile ground for healing and vitality.

As research continues to unravel the complexities of DMSO, we may witness a shift in its perception and application. Further investigations may shed light on its mechanisms of action, validate its effectiveness for various conditions, and refine its usage guidelines.

It's conceivable that DMSO's future may involve more targeted applications, perhaps in combination with other therapies or as a delivery system for enhancing the efficacy of existing medications. The scientific community's ongoing exploration of DMSO holds the promise of unlocking its full potential and harnessing its power for therapeutic benefit.

In the end, the decision to explore DMSO rests in your hands. Armed with the knowledge you've gained from this book, you're better equipped to navigate the complexities, weigh the potential benefits and risks, and engage in informed conversations with your healthcare provider.

If you choose to embark on the DMSO journey, do so with a discerning mind, a spirit of curiosity, and an unwavering commitment to your well-being. Remember, your health is a precious asset, and it deserves the utmost care and consideration.

While this book has provided a comprehensive overview of DMSO, it's merely a starting point. The world of health and wellness is vast and ever-evolving. Continue to seek knowledge, explore diverse perspectives, and cultivate a lifelong commitment to learning and self-discovery.

Embrace the wisdom of both conventional and alternative approaches, and remain open to new possibilities. Your health journey is unique, and it's an ongoing process of exploration, adaptation, and growth.

As we conclude this exploration of DMSO, let us remember that true healing is a multi-faceted journey. It encompasses not only the physical body but also the mind and spirit. It's a journey of self-discovery, resilience, and the unwavering pursuit of well-being.

May this book serve as a guide, a source of information, and a catalyst for informed action. May it empower you to take an active role in your health, to make choices that align with your values, and to cultivate a life of vitality and purpose.

***Thank you for joining us on this journey into the world of DMSO. May your path be filled with knowledge, wisdom, and unwavering well-being.***

www.ingramcontent.com/pod-product-compliance
Lightning Source LLC
Chambersburg PA
CBHW071653240526
45469CB00021B/2276